Ebola and Marburg Viruses

A View of Infection Using Electron Microscopy

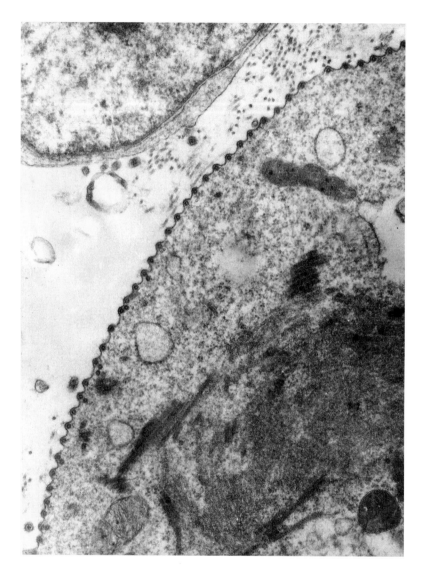

Photograph of a chick embryo infected with Ebola virus, as seen using an electron microscope. A viral inclusion, the factory for reproducing Ebola virions, is obvious as a dark body with dark linear nucleocapsids. Some Ebola nucleocapsids have traveled to the cell membrane and are budding from the surface. Once they leave the cell, the Ebola viruses are ready to travel and infect other cells. These free Ebola viruses can be seen between the two cells. (Magnification 26,000)

On the cover, the upper part of the image shown above is interpreted in color by computer artistry. The coloring does *not* represent that of the actual microscope image.

Ebola and Marburg Viruses

A View of Infection Using Electron Microscopy

ELENA I. RYABCHIKOVA, PH.D.

AND

BARBARA B. S. PRICE, PH.D.

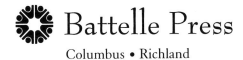

Battelle Press

Columbus • Richland

Library of Congress Cataloging-in-Publication Data

Ryabchikova, Elena, 1951–
    Ebola and Marburg viruses : a view of infection using electron
  microscopy / Elena Ryabchikova and Barbara B.S. Price.
      p. ; cm
    Includes bibliographical references and index.
    ISBN 1-57477-131-0 (case bound : alk. paper)
      1. Ebola virus disease—Pathogenesis. 2. Marburg virus disease—
  Pathogenesis. 3. Electron microscopy. I. Price, Barbara B.S., 1945–
  II. Title.
      [DNLM: 1. Filoviridae Infections—pathology. 2. Filoviridae—
  pathogenicity. 3. Microscopy, Electron. WC 501 R988e 2002]
  QR201.E16 R97 2002
    616.9′25—dc21   2002066732

Printed in the United States of America

Although the authors have had the support of both Vector and Battelle,
the opinions and views expressed in this book are those of the authors
and do not necessarily state or reflect those of Vector, Battelle, the
Russian government, the U.S. Government, or any agency thereof.

Battelle Press
505 King Avenue
Columbus, Ohio 43201
Phone: 1-800-451-3543 or 614-424-6393
Fax: 614-424-3819
E-mail: press@battelle.org
Web bookstore: www.battelle.org/bookstore

Dedication

To
MARIA SERGEEVNA VINOGRADOVA,
Professor at the Novosibirsk State University in Russia.
She has been my teacher, good friend, and
supporter in all my professional endeavors.
E. I. R.

To
RICHARD MAYER PRICE.
I would never have attempted this
without his support and encouragement.
B. B. S. P.

Acknowledgements

This book took several years to put together, during which time many people contributed to the project, some with financial support, some with actual work, and some with emotional and moral support. The authors lived more than 12,000 km from each other; for communication purposes they took advantage of e-mail and scientific conferences, especially the Chemical Biological Medical Treatment Symposia (CBMTS) series initiated and operated by Applied Science and Analysis (ASA), Inc.

Dr. Elena I. Ryabchikova, with the help of other scientists and technicians, performed all the experiments. They were conducted at SRC VB Vector, where she had the support of Professor Lev S. Sandakhchiev, Director General of Vector and Fellow of the Russian Academy of Science, and Professor Sergey Netesov, Deputy Director General of Vector and Director of the Molecular Biology Institute. The authors thank in particular Drs. Ju. Rassadkin, A. Shestopalov, A. Sergeev, and S. Luchko, and their co-workers at Vector. Dr. Ryabchikova also extends many thanks to all employees of the Laboratory of Ultrastructural Investigations and Pathomorphology.

The many international scientists who helped with the filoviral studies included, in particular, Dr. S. Becker at the Institute of Virology (Marburg, Germany); he conducted the time course studies of filoviral infection in Vero cells. Those studies were supported by the International Association for Cooperation with Scientists from the former Soviet Union (INTAS) (Grants #96-1361 and #99-00750).

Dr. Barbara B. S. Price worked with Dr. Ryabchikova to help her express her ideas in English and organize the results of her experiments into a form appropriate for publishing. In this work, Dr. Price had the support of ASA, Inc., and Battelle Memorial Institute, where she especially appreciated the technical editing skills and patience of Karla Uttenreither Mack. Dr. Price extends her thanks also to Dr. Katherine M. Byrne for her internal review and to Dr. David M. Robinson for his internal review and continued support.

Both authors express their gratitude to Drs. Nancy Jaax and Thomas Geisbert for their very thorough external reviews and thoughtful comments.

Clearly, international effort and cooperation were crucial to this book's success in describing the advantages of using electron microscopy to understand filoviral infections.

Contents

Figures and Tables

> NOTE: In the photographs accompanying the text, numbers and an adjacent legend identify pertinent items. For the sake of clarity, when there are several items that illustrate the same subject, only a few examples are identified.

FIGURES

TABLES

Preface

Electron microscopy occupies a special position among the techniques for viral research. Unlike a light microscope, the electron microscope is a sophisticated, expensive instrument that requires highly qualified and trained scientists to successfully operate it and interpret the results. Techniques for sample preparation, and for the actual microscopic examination, are complex and must be followed precisely. "A jeweler's work is coarse by comparison," as D.C. Pease noted in the preface to *Histological Techniques for Electron Microscopy* (1960). Nevertheless, the technique of electron microscopy is widely and effectively used in viral research and in rapid diagnosis of viral diseases of man and animals.

Since viruses with particle diameters of only 20–300 nm are beyond the resolving capacity of the light microscope, the electron microscope has become the unique tool to view and study the physical aspects of viral replication within the cell. Although D. Ivanovsky discovered the tobacco mosaic virus in 1892, the physical characteristics of the virus were unknown for the next 50 years. In 1940, the first electron micrograph of a virus, that of vaccinia virus, was published [Ruska, 1940]. Although the early pictures of vaccinia virus failed to portray the shape and size of the viral particles as they occurred in aqueous solutions [Williams,

1953], they provided tangible evidence for the existence of viruses. The electron microscope allowed scientists to peer into the universe of the cell and eventually that of the virus. "It has become evident that the electron microscope is peculiarly appealing in its ability to present us with direct information regarding virus morphology" [Williams, 1953]. As methods for diagnosing and identifying viruses by electron microscopy underwent intensive development in the 1960s and 1970s, images from the electron microscope established that the sizes and the intermediate and final structures of virions formed during their replication in cells are specific to each family and genus. Certain morphological features of the viruses, as with other forms of life, are now regarded as identifiable and are included in virus classifications. With the development of new techniques applicable to electron microscopy and with improvements in sample preparations, the physical characteristics of new viruses have been described. No one had ever thought that the universe of the viruses would contain such a variety of features and shapes—such strange sights viewed in the electron microscopic images had not been expected. Viruses were shaped as spheres and icosahedrons, rods and bricks, cylinders and bullets. Even structures on and in viruses could be seen, such as minute spikes of different lengths, jutting from the virus' surface.

Each virus family has its peculiar structural and functional attributes of undeniable interest. However, attention is still focused on viruses that are pathogenic and lethal. Among these pathogenic viruses are Ebola and Marburg. They have become notorious because of their fulminant disease course, high mortality, and the failure of scientists to find a vaccine or an effective treatment. Furthermore, Ebola and Marburg viruses are perceived as mysterious because their natural reservoirs have not been discovered. Other viral, bacterial, and parasitic diseases (e.g., AIDS, dysentery, malaria, etc.) threaten populations in developing countries of Africa and South America; however, none of these diseases have captured the public's imagination, as have Ebola and Marburg viruses.

Occasionally, a single book is able to draw together seemingly isolated events and invite the public to approach a topic with a new level of synthesis and discussion. One such book is

R. Preston's *The Hot Zone* (1994) about the emerging filoviruses and their implications to virology. The film *Outbreak* is loosely based on *The Hot Zone* and is as thought provoking as the book, despite the film's sensationalism. It is clear that Preston was fascinated by the subject and became knowledgeable about virology. On a different plane, *Level 4: Virus Hunters of the CDC* (1996), written by J. McCormick (one of the discoverers of the filoviruses) and S. Fisher-Hoch, includes an authoritative account of the history of the filoviruses. The filoviruses are only a few of the many agents causing severe diseases whose popularization may lead to accelerated research and a better understanding of the disease process. However, by revealing the nature of viral infections, studies of filoviruses have contributed and continue to contribute to the advancement of virology as a fundamental biological science.

The results of many years of research conducted in the Laboratory of Ultrastructural Investigations and Pathomorphology (LUIP) of the State Research Center of Virology and Biotechnology Vector (SRC VB Vector) in Koltsovo, the Novosibirsk region, Russia, amply support the idea that the natures of Ebola and Marburg viruses are unique. We found that in the course of lethal infection, the filoviruses not only attack and damage their preferential targets (blood clotting system, liver, and kidneys), but they also profoundly affect the organs of the immune and hematopoietic systems. The immune system fails to discriminate filovirus-infected cells and lacks the immune response to counter the infection in an effective manner. Evidence indicates that crucial events during filoviral infections unfold in the bloodstream and that successful infection of the macrophage is the initial critical event. The results obtained through the research conducted at LUIP and other sections of SRC VB Vector have helped to develop a concept for the pathogenesis of filoviral hemorrhagic fevers, a concept that is suggested as a vantage point for future interpretations.

This book attempts to consolidate the recent literature, published and unpublished, and the author's (E.I.R.) insight (developed over 30 years of electron microscopy and virology studies) to tell the story of filoviruses and how they invade and conquer their hosts (i.e., the pathogenesis of the diseases they cause). This book describes the overall, dynamic properties of the virus. We attempt to follow the stages of filoviral infection from the individual cell to the greater unit of the whole organism. Based on a survey of the literature and our data, we offer a current scheme that reconstructs the sequential events that occur in filoviral infections.

This book also seeks to demonstrate the quality and usefulness of work that can be done with the electron microscope in studies of viral infections and pathological processes. The electron microscope is critical to the study of viruses and should be integrated into experimental designs, including studies on the pathogenesis of viral infections.

And finally, we hope to write lucidly for investigators in the widely diversified fields of medicine and biology. The book is addressed to this group, and for this reason, some terms and concepts are redefined for those not familiar with virology jargon. The book is designed to inform virologists about the electron microscope. By incorporating electron microscopy with traditional methods of research, virologists will have the opportunity to correlate and expand data and bridge information gaps.

In 1987, Nermut expressed the hope "that in the next decade a more comprehensive understanding of the structure of all viruses will be obtained which will be of benefit to both general and medical virology" [Nermut, 1987]. We place hope in our book as an attempt to achieve a comprehensive understanding of the replication and ultrastructural pathogenesis of the filoviruses.

Ebola and Marburg Viruses

A View of Infection Using Electron Microscopy

chapter 1

Introduction

Virology is the study of viruses and viral diseases. Viruses, and the special class of filoviruses, represent just one of the many causes of morbidity and mortality in humans. For commonality in terms, this chapter briefly discusses viruses, filoviruses, and a review of the history of filoviruses.

Viruses and Virology

Hundreds of different viruses have been discovered. There are viruses that uniquely attack fungi, plants, insects, amphibians, reptiles, birds, and mammals. Insights into the parasitic nature of viruses, regardless of the particular virus type, are valuable since knowledge gained from studying these smallest living forms at the ultracellular level enables us to better understand their interaction patterns at many levels, including virus-human interactions.

Viruses are composed of either deoxyribose nucleic acid (DNA) or ribose nucleic acid (RNA). All viruses are obligate parasites, which means they must use the host cell's mechanisms to reproduce; viruses cannot reproduce by themselves and with rare exceptions, the DNA or RNA do not contain the genetic codes for enzymes. A fully assembled virus is called a virion. The virion consists most simply of the genome (either DNA or RNA) protected by a protein coat, called a capsid, which may be further protected by an envelope made of a membrane of glycoproteins and lipids. The capsid and nucleic acid together are called the nucleocapsid. Some viruses acquire the envelope from the cellular membranes of the host cell during budding from the cell and are called "enveloped viruses," while other viruses have no membrane envelope.

In virology, "isolate," "clone," and "strain" are commonly used to differentiate between viruses isolated from different sources. A "viral (virus) isolate" is a sample containing the living virus, which was obtained from a single host. No special characterization of the virus' biological properties is implied in relation to a viral isolate. Many viral isolates may be obtained during one outbreak because each new host (human, animal, or vector) means a new isolate. Isolates may differ in their biological properties. A "viral (virus) clone" is a viral preparation derived from one viral particle and presumed to have identical genetic characteristics. A "viral (virus) strain" is a viral preparation characterized by some parameters (e.g., ability to infect animals or cell cultures, resistance to chemicals, etc.).

When discussing viruses, the terms "infection" and "disease" are often used. In this book, we have attempted to differentiate between the terms. Infection is the term used when the virus replicates in a cell, tissue, or organ, and the term is also used to describe manifestations or effects that result directly from the infection. Disease is the collection of symptoms, especially those that are an indirect result of the infection (e.g., the change in endothelial cell permeability that results from the release of cytokines from an infected cell).

The SRC VB Vector has been studying the biological properties of a great number of viruses: the human immunodeficiency virus, measles, mumps, influenza, encephalitis, hepatitis A, B, and C, and poxviruses, among others. The molecular-biological characteristics, infection specificity in animals, and viral reproduction in cell culture are all under study. The goal is to develop diagnostic procedures for viruses, vaccines, and anti-viral drug therapies. The analysis of the developmental mechanisms of viral infections, notably Marburg and Ebola, is part of the fundamental investigations of Vector.

The LUIP has been working on viruses and studying their reproduction in cell culture and animals for more than 15 years. The emphasis of these studies is the use of light and electron microscopy to investigate the pathogenic mechanisms of viral infections. Most of these studies have been published in Russian journals; recently, more of the work has been published in English in international journals. Researchers from LUIP made the first direct observation using electron microscopy that the Venezuelan equine encephalitis virus migrates along the olfactory nerve from the nasal cavity to the brain, bypassing the bloodstream [Ryzhikov, 1995]. Another observation came from Kochneva and Serpinski, researchers who obtained data showing that mousepox viruses deficient in the gene for thymidine kinase lose their pathogenicity for the mouse host [Kochneva, 1994; Serpinski, 1996]. However, the major research focus in the LUIP remains the pathogenesis of filoviral infections. (For a comprehensive review of the results obtained by the LUIP, the reader is referred to *Animal Pathology of Filoviral Infections* [Ryabchikova, 1999] and other sources referenced therein.)

Experimental virology is at an important stage; viral infectious diseases can be modeled based on pathogenesis (mechanisms of the disease development) and the immune response of the host. These models can then be used to explore therapies for the disease produced by the viral infection. The choice of the appropriate model is a very important task for virologists. Not all viruses can be modeled to obtain experimental data comparable to human infections. Higher primates are frequently the only suitable models for infection (e.g., measles, hepatitis, and tick-borne encephalitis), but their use in experiments is often limited. Fortunately, the filoviruses can be modeled in non-human primates and some of the pathogenic effects also can be modeled in guinea pigs. The experimental studies on pathogenesis are valuable because the underlying causes and clinical manifestations of viral diseases are common to many viruses. For example, understanding the development of blood system damage resulting from the derangement of blood clotting in filoviral diseases can be useful in analyzing other viral hemorrhagic fevers (VHFs). There are four families (or groups) of viruses that cause viral hemorrhagic fevers:

Family	Genus	VHFs
Filoviridae	"Ebola-like" *Filovirus* "Marburg-like" *Filovirus*	Ebola Marburg
Bunyaviridae	*Hantavirus* *Nairovirus*	Hantaan Crimean Congo
Flaviviridae	*Flavivirus*	Dengue
Arenaviridae	*Arenavirus*	Lassa

Filoviruses

Modern concepts of filoviral pathology are predominately based on early experimental studies, which were designed to identify and characterize these new viral agents. These experiments were necessarily searching for the unique features in filoviruses. Data addressing the pathogenic mechanisms and features common to the filoviruses are scarce. This is particularly true for data that address the development of disease because the incubation period is so short. While there are many excellent resources for information about filoviral epidemiology, few descriptions of animal studies exist. For a comprehensive review of all published data in all branches of filovirology, the reader is urged to see *The Filoviruses*, Editor Prof. H.D. Klenk [Current Topics in Microbiology and Immunology, 235, 1999]. The chapter "Animal Pathology of Filoviral Infections" [Ryabchikova, 1999] summarizes all of the published data on filoviral pathology in animals through 1996. Regretfully, a broader presentation of our results pertinent to filoviral pathogenesis was beyond the scope of *The Filoviruses*.

The results of many years of research conducted in the LUIP amply support the unique nature of Marburg and Ebola viruses. During the course of a lethal infection, the filoviruses not only attack and damage their main targets, the blood circulation system and the liver, but they also profoundly affect the organs of the immune system and hemopoiesis. The immune system fails to use either specific immune cells or unspecific immune response to identify the filovirus-infected cells. Our evidence indicates that infection of macrophages triggers filoviral pathogenesis, and the crucial events during filoviral infections occur in the bloodstream and lymphatics. The results support a conceptual model for the pathogenesis of filoviral hemorrhagic fevers; we propose this model as a vantage point for future interpretations.

In virology, all findings that can be used to explain how damage to various organs develops are important. Our studies were devoted mainly to the examination of filoviral replication and pathological changes during the course of the fatal infection. We also performed comparative studies of fatal filoviral infections primarily to establish common features, which may be useful for understanding the mechanisms of filoviral disease development. With this in mind, we designed our experiments so that they would reproduce a pathological process, mimicking the process in humans as close as possible. Thereby, we hoped to obtain data that would explain the developmental mechanisms of the disease from which concepts for therapeutic intervention could be derived. For this reason, we analyzed the time course of disease by using infectious doses of the virus in concentrations that might be expected in natural exposures. The details of filoviruses' structure and function, their roles in infection of cell cultures, and intact animal models are the subjects of this book.

Filoviruses: A Review of Their History

The history of infectious diseases is marked by recurrent, intermittent outbreaks of newly emerging diseases. However, due to modern transportation and worldwide contacts, it is now possible for these diseases to generate worldwide epidemics, known as pandemics. Filoviral infections are examples of highly pathogenic emerging viral diseases. Based on their biological properties and the lack of protective vaccines and effective drug treatments, the filoviruses were classified by the World Health Organization (WHO) as pathogens requiring the maximum biosafety level, P4 (an older designation that is similar to BSL-4) [BMBL, 1993; WHO, 1985].

In 1967, "primary" outbreaks of unknown hemorrhagic fever occurred at about the same time in Germany (Marburg and Frankfurt) and Yugoslavia (Belgrade). This disease affected laboratory workers who had contact with monkey blood and tissues. Additional cases involved relatives of the victims and their health care providers. In all, 31 cases occurred, including six secondary infections and seven deaths [Draper, 1977; Siegert, 1967]. The blood and organs of these patients were inoculated into guinea pigs and cell cultures and a virus was isolated. The disease was called Marburg hemorrhagic fever and the virus was named the Marburg virus (also known as Marburg disease virus). The morphology of the Marburg virus was unique and the virus was antigenically unrelated to any other known human pathogen [Kissling, 1968; Smith, 1967]. After these first outbreaks, the Marburg virus disappeared until 1975, when three cases of Marburg hemorrhagic fever were recorded in Johannesburg, South Africa. The index patient was a man who had traveled in Zimbabwe before contracting hemorrhagic fever; he died after a 12-day course of infection. The other two subjects recovered [Gear, 1975; Rippey, 1976]. Single fatal cases of Marburg hemorrhagic fever were recorded in Kenya in 1980 and in 1987. Investigations were conducted to identify natural reservoirs in the African regions where the index cases appeared. A cave inhabited by bats stirred interest because a victim had visited it shortly before becoming ill. However, in all the studies, no evidence of the natural reservoir of Marburg virus has yet been discovered [Feldmann, 1996a; Peters, 1991]. The total number of humans who have had disease following infection with the Marburg virus is 37, of which nine cases were fatal [WHO, 1985].

Two closely related viruses, causing epidemics of severe hemorrhagic fever in Zaire and Sudan in 1976, were isolated and named the Ebola virus (Ebola-Zaire and Ebola-Sudan). More than 550 cases were reported; of these cases, more than 430 were fatal. Although morphologically similar, the viruses were serologically distinct from the Marburg virus. The Ebola virus could spread by close contact with the patients in hospitals. Syringes and needles reused after contact with Ebola viral hemorrhagic fever patients also spread the virus to others. In 1977 and 1979, two outbreaks of Ebola viral hemorrhagic fever were reported in Zaire (now the

Democratic Republic of the Congo) and Sudan [Bowen, 1977; WHO, 1978; WHO 1978a]. In 1989, a filoviral disease was reported in a primate import quarantine facility in Reston, Virginia (USA). The responsible virus, identified as an isolate of Ebola virus, Ebola Reston, resulted in numerous deaths in cynomolgus monkeys imported from the Philippines. The virus did not produce disease in the workers in the facility; however, some seroconversion did occur [Jahrling, 1990; CDC, 1990]. Genomic sequence analyses of the viruses have shown that Ebola virus Reston and African Ebola virus (Sudan and Zaire) originated from independent sources [Feldmann, 1999a; Ikegami, 2001]. An identical isolate of the Ebola viruses was found in a monkey facility in Pennsylvania [Hayes, 1992; Jahrling, 1990]. An epidemic of Ebola in the Tai Forest of Cote d'Ivoire in 1994 killed a number of chimpanzees [Formenty, 1999a]. The Cote d'Ivoire outbreak also infected a Swiss primatologist, who was evacuated back to Switzerland and survived with intensive medical intervention and management [Formenty, 1999; LeGuenno, 1995].

Cases of Ebola virus fever have continued to emerge sporadically. The latest outbreaks were recorded in Gabon in 1996, in Uganda in 2001, and in Gabon and the Democratic Republic of the Congo in February 2002. Ebola continues to be identified in the Congo region. As of 14 April 2003, ProMed (www.promedmail.org) reported 140 cases, including 123 deaths in humans in the latest outbreak. The outbreak is believed to have been caused by villagers eating primates which were already infected with Ebola [ProMed-mail, 5 Feb 2003]. Also 600–800 western lowland gorillas are believed to have died as a result of Ebola infections in the Democratic Republic of the Congo [ProMed-mail, 4 April 2003].

The mortality rates for the 1995 and 1996 outbreaks were 78% and 66%, respectively [MMWR, 1995; Georges, 1996]. The causative agent was established as belonging to the Zaire subtype of Ebola virus. The analysis of the viral nucleotide sequence in the Gabon isolate showed extensive homology to the Kikwit-95 isolate of the Ebola-Zaire virus. Further analysis showed that both viral isolates (Kikwit-95 and the Gabon-96) seem to have evolved from a progenitor virus different from that of the Zaire-76 isolates. This is a different strain from any of the Zaire virus isolates obtained at different geographical locations over a period of 20 years. The high degree of similarity between the Zaire, Kikwit, and Gabon strains and the lack of similarity to isolates from other locations over 20 years demonstrate an extreme conservation of the genome in the as yet unknown natural reservoir of Ebola virus [Volchkov, 1997].

There have been more than 23 Marburg and Ebola virus outbreaks among humans and monkeys since 1967; these outbreaks have affected more than 1,100 people [Schou, 2000]. One of the recent outbreaks of filoviral disease occurred in the Durba region located in the northeastern part of the Democratic Republic of the Congo. The causative agent was identified as the Marburg virus. Sixty of the 73 people infected died, which corresponds to 82% mortality and is identical to previously measured Ebola-Zaire virus mortality. This outbreak was the first of Marburg virus disease not involving laboratory contamination. Initial epidemiologic findings suggest that the first cases involved gold miners who were probably infected by contact with an animal reservoir such as bats [Bertherat, 1999].

Filoviruses: Taxonomy

Both Ebola and Marburg viruses are filoviruses and are in the *Filoviridae* family of the order Mononegavirales. The *Filoviridae* family was named for the presence of rod-like, or more accurately, filamentous-shaped viral particles [Kiley, 1982]. Each enveloped filovirus has a genome composed of a single molecule of negative-sense single-stranded RNA, about 19 kb in size. We will explore the structures in more detail in Chapter 4 of this book. According to the latest decision of the International Committee on Taxonomy of Viruses (ICTV) in 2002, the *Filoviridae* family includes two genera, "Marburg-like viruses" and "Ebola-like viruses" [http://www.ncbi.nlm.nih.gov/ICTVdb/Ictv/index.htm, updated 19 January 2002]. *Marburg virus* (MARV) is the only species in the Marburg-like viruses and six strains are listed: Musoke, Ratayczak, Popp, Voege, Ozolin, and Marburg Ravn. The Ebola-like genera consists of four viral species: *Cote d'Ivoire Ebola virus* (CIEBOV) with one strain (Cote d'Ivoire), *Reston Ebola virus* (REBOV) with four strains (Reston, Philippines, Siena, and Texas), *Sudan Ebola virus* (SEBOV) with two strains (Boniface and Maleo), and *Zaire Ebola virus* (ZEBOV) with six strains

(Mayinga, Zaire, Eckron, Tandala, Kikwit, and Gabon). Older reports may use different acronyms for the species and may not list the strains using this nomenclature. For the sake of clarity in our studies that we report on here, we used MARV (strain Popp) and ZEBOV (strain Zaire, 1976). When comparing our data with other studies, it is important to remember that differences in filovirus species, and even the strains, can give different results depending on which aspect of the virus' properties are being investigated. If it is clear which Ebola virus species was used in other work, we will note that; otherwise, we will use a generic notation of EBOV for Ebola viruses.

chapter 2

Materials and Methods

All experimental studies were performed in the Institute of Molecular Biology, State Research Center of Virology and Biotechnology Vector (SRC VB Vector), Russian Ministry of Public Health (Koltsovo, Novosibirsk Region). Experiments with living Marburg virus (MARV) and Ebola virus (ZEBOV), and preparation of the samples of filovirus-infected animals and cells, for both light and electron microscopic studies, were performed in special facilities with maximal P4 level of biosafety by Drs. Ju. Rassadkin, A. Shestopalov, A. Sergeev, S. Luchko, and their co-workers. Dr. S. Becker in the Institute of Virology (Marburg, Germany) conducted the time course studies of filoviral infection in Vero cells; these studies were supported by INTAS (Grants #96-1361 and # 99-00750).

Viruses

MARV (strain Popp), passaged six times in guinea pigs, was obtained from the Institute of Poliomyelitis and Viral Encephalitidies (Russia). The virus stock was a 10% suspension of the liver of guinea pigs at the seventh passage with a titer of 10^7 LD_{50} for guinea pigs by the intraperitoneal (IP) route. The suspension was prepared in Eagle's minimal essential medium (MEM), supplemented with 2% bovine sera and antibiotics.

ZEBOV, passaged twice in green monkeys (strain Zaire, 1976), was provided by the Department of Virology, Institute of Microbiology (Ministry of Defense, Russia). The virus stock was a 10% suspension of green monkey liver, at the third passage, with a titer of $10^{7.5}$ LD_{50}, as determined by serial 10-fold dilutions of liver homogenate samples intracerebrally (IC) injected into newborn mice; calculated by the Spearman-Kaerber method. The liver was obtained from monkeys euthanized at day 5 post-inoculation, before development of necrotic processes to avoid contamination of the viral stock by endotoxins. The suspension was prepared in Eagle's MEM solution with 2% bovine sera and antibiotic supplements [Ryabchikova, 1999a]. Viral stocks were prepared at SRC VB Vector and stored at -70 °C until use.

Animals and Cell Cultures

The animals used were outbred adult guinea pigs (250–300 g), outbred newborn mice (aged less than 24 h), outbred adult mice, adult male Chinchilla rabbits (2.5 kg), green monkeys (*Cercopitecus aethiops*), rhesus monkeys (*Macaca mulatta*), baboons (*Papio hamadryas*), and cynomolgus monkeys (*Macaca fascicularis*). Vero cells and L-68 (human diploid cells) were used. The animals and cells were obtained from the Department of Experimental Animals and Institute of Cell Cultures of SRC VB Vector, Russia. The Vero cells used by Dr. Becker in studies in Marburg, Germany were E-6 clone cells. All animal experiments were designed and conducted under Russian animal experimentation ethics regulations. Animals were anesthetized before handling.

Table 2-1 describes the filoviral experiments in animals that provided the samples for our microscopic studies. There are two major points to be made in Table 2-1. The first point is critical to understanding our experiments and our results, especially when comparing them to experiments done at other laboratories. In most of our experiments, we used extremely low doses of virus in order to allow the animals a chance to develop their defensive measures. Most of the other experiments reported in the literature

Table 2-1. Description of the filoviral experiments in animals that provided the samples for microscopic studies.

Goal of the Experiment	Animal Species (number)	Infectious Dose/ Inoculation Mode	Tissue Sampling
Studies of Marburg virus reproduction and pathological changes in visceral organs[1,2]	Guinea pigs (26)	100 LD_{50}[*]/ IP[†]	3 animals for LM[‡] and EM[§], daily. 2 animals were injected with saline (control) and euthanized on day 8 post-inoculation.
Studies of Marburg virus reproduction and pathological changes in visceral organs[3]	Guinea pigs (40)	2–5 LD_{50}/ aerosol	3 animals for LM and EM, daily. Total of 27 animals and 3 controls. 10 of the animals were used for preparation of the lavage for examining the alveolar macrophages.
Studies of Marburg virus reproduction and pathological changes in visceral organs[1,2]	Green monkeys (9)	100 LD_{50}/ IP	1 animal for LM and EM, daily. 2 monkeys were euthanized on days 6 and 7.
Studies of Ebola virus reproduction and pathological changes in visceral organs in nonlethal infection[4]	Guinea pigs (42)	10^5 LD_{50} for newborn mice/IP	3 animals for LM and EM, on days 3, 5, 7, 9, 11, 12, 13, 15, 18, 21, 24, 26, and 28. 3 control animals were euthanized on day 28.
Examination of the infection changes during sequential passages of Ebola virus[4]	Guinea pigs (44)	1 mL 10% liver homogenate from animals on previous passage/IP	Day 7 after inoculation, from 3 animals of each of 8 passages. From 3–4 animals on days 5 and 8 at passages 5, 6, and 7.

continued

Table 2-1. Description of the filoviral experiments in animals that provided the samples for microscopic studies *(continued)*

Goal of the Experiment	Animal Species (number)	Infectious Dose/ Inoculation Mode	Tissue Sampling
Examine the spread of Ebola from the injection site over time[5]	Guinea pigs (10)	200 LD_{50}/IM[‖]	1, 2, 4, 12 h after SC injection, from 1 animal each time; 24, 36, and 48 h after SC injection, from 2 animals each time.
Time course studies of Ebola virus reproduction and pathological changes in visceral organs[6]	Green monkeys (12)	100 LD_{50}/SC[#]	Days 1–4, 1 animal; day 5, 3 animals; days 6–7, 2 animals, day 8, 1 animal.
Comparative studies of Ebola virus reproduction and pathological changes in visceral organs after different inoculation modes	Green monkeys (20)	100 LD_{50}/via 4 modes: IP, SC, intratracheal, and via gastric tube into stomach	At the terminal stages from all 16 animals for LM and EM. 4 monkeys were used for each inoculation route, and 4 monkeys were injected with saline for control.
Examination of Ebola virus reproduction and pathological changes in visceral organs[6]	Baboons (13)	20–50 LD_{50}/SC	At the terminal stages from all animals for LM and EM.
Examination of species-specific differences in Ebola virus reproduction and pathological changes in visceral organs[5]	Green monkeys (4) Rhesus monkeys (4) Baboons (4) Cynomolgus monkeys (4)	1–10 LD_{50}/SC	At the terminal stages from all animals for LM and EM.

[*]LD_{50} – lethal dose (LD) of agent required to kill 50% of test animals in one dose
[†]IP – intraperitoneal
[‡]LM – light microscopy
[§]EM – electron microscopy
[‖]IM – intramuscular
[#]SC – subcutaneous—injection in mice/guinea pigs given in the upper part of the hip; injection in monkeys given in upper part of the arm

[1] Ryabchikova, 1994
[2] Skripchenko, 1994
[3] Ryabchikova, 1996a
[4] Ryabchikova, 1996
[5] Ryabchikova, 1998
[6] Ryabchikova, 1999

used much higher doses in which the animals died and, in fact, the changes observed in the organs were very uniform because the virus infection completely overwhelmed the animals. In a few experiments, we used higher doses, 1000 LD_{50} and 10^5 LD_{50}, so that we could compare our results with others.

The second point is that we looked at six different modes of inoculation: intraperitoneal (injection into the peritoneal cavity), intramuscular (injection into the muscle), subcutaneous (injection under the skin), intratracheal (injection into the trachea), inhalation of aerosol, and directly into the stomach via gastric tube. As noted in Table 2-1, we performed several experiments specifically to compare different inoculation modes. Different inoculation modes were also used on the animals, including at various infectious doses, to simulate the different possible routes of infection. Details of the virological experiments are described in the publications noted in the table.

The biological activities of MARV and ZEBOV were determined by two methods: by plaque-forming units (PFU) on Vero cells under an agar overlay, and by titration in IC-inoculated newborn mice (ZEBOV) or IP-infected guinea pigs (MARV). ZEBOV and MARV reproduction and pathological changes were studied in visceral organs, including the liver, kidney, lungs, and spleen. These are the organs that have the greatest contact with blood and lymph. If a virus is carried by blood, we would expect to see the largest concentrations of virus in these visceral organs.

Samples for light and electron microscopic studies were taken from the anesthetized guinea pigs and monkeys in time course studies or immediately after animal death (terminal stages of the infection). The specific conditions for infecting animals and cell cultures are given in Chapter 4.

Electron Microscopy Sample Preparation

Tissue specimens were dissected from liver, spleen, kidney, adrenal glands, lungs, peritracheal area, trachea, tracheal bifurcation, peribronchial, mesenteric and inguinal lymph nodes, bone marrow, and intestines. All samples were fixed in 4% paraformaldehyde, post-fixed in 1% osmium tetraoxide in Hank's solution, dehydrated according to standard techniques, and embedded in an Epon-Araldite mixture. Cell preparations were first centrifuged for 5 min at 3,000–5,000 revolutions/min and the pellets were fixed as above. Embedded samples were sliced in Reichert-Jung ultramicrotomes (Austria) using glass knives; semithin and ultrathin sections were prepared.

Semithin sections for light microscopy were stained with Azure 2. Areas for electron microscopic examinations were selected in the semithin sections of the organs under the light microscope. In each animal, at least three samples of each organ were examined at three levels. Such sampling is very important because it reduces mistakes in evaluating electron microscopic observations. Indeed, only small areas may be examined in the electron microscope (about 1000 μm [1mm] by 700–800 μm). If a researcher does not select the particular small area under the light microscope (usually from 100 to 500 magnification), it is possible to miss an area of important details or to make erroneous conclusions based on unique observations. It is necessary to determine how regular or unique the observation is at the light microscope level and then examine the small area or the ultrastructure with the electron microscope.

Ultrathin sections were stained with uranyl acetate and lead citrate. Sections were examined using JEM-100S (Jeol, Japan) and H600 (Hitachi, Japan) microscopes. Ultrathin sectioning provides good electron microscopic images, with sharp details of the internal structures of the cells and virions (Figure 2-1). The changes in tissues occurring during viral infections were followed by examinations of the ultrathin sections.

In general, small viruses have a complex three-dimensional structure that is observable only in the electron microscope. Negative staining is widely used in virus research and diagnostics because viruses can be detected faster with this method than with other available techniques. A drop of virus-containing material is first applied onto a coated formvar (modified polyvinyl acetal resins) or colloidion (highly purified nitrocellulose) supporting film, and then the contrast material is added. Heavy metal salts, phosphotungstate, or uranyl acetate, are used as contrast material [Nermut, 1987]. These electron-dense salts surround the viral particles, making their contours conspicuous. The contrast materials penetrate into the virions to different depths, thereby revealing the surface and parts of the internal structures. The results are bright viral particles against a dark background (Figure 2-2). For

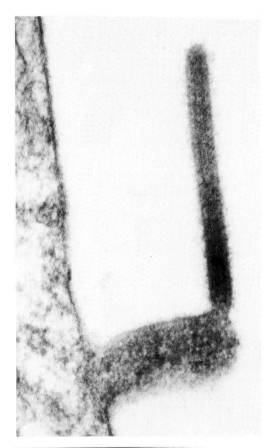

Figure 2-1. An electron microscope photograph of MARV made from an ultrathin section (magnification 87,500). The cell and the viral particle are dark on a light background.

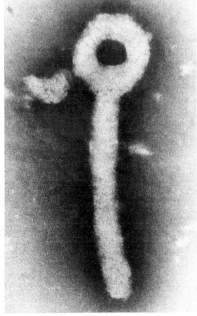

Figure 2-2. An electron microscope picture of MARV particles negatively stained by uranyl acetate (magnification 120,000). The viral particles appear light on a dark background.

this reason, this technique for the visualization of viral particles is called negative staining. Detection and identification of viruses in various virus-containing fluids, including blood and body fluids from clinical patients, can be done with negative staining. Negative staining is helpful in studies of viral shape and surface. Its disadvantage is its limited sensitivity; in order to successfully detect the viruses in a sample, 1 mL of the sample should contain at least 1,000,000 (10^6) viral particles. In our studies, we used negative staining for examining the viral preparations from the blood of infected animals and tissue culture media. Typically, the concentration of viral particles was 10^7–10^8 particles/mL.

Summary

Careful preparation of the samples containing viral particles is essential to following the course of infection of viruses. By combining various preparation and photographic techniques, an experienced electron microscopist can bring the very small world of viruses out of the realm of pictorial curiosities to a more sophisticated study of the cause and course of a viral disease.

chapter 3

Morphology of Filoviruses

Filoviral Shapes

The investigators who first examined a negatively stained Marburg virus (MARV) suspension in an electron microscope [Korb, 1969; Peters, 1969] were astounded by the great variety of shapes they saw. The MARV particles were present as rods of different lengths, 6-shaped structures, pleomorphic structures, and branched rods (containing branches either in the middle or at both ends). These MARV particles were morphologically different (and more polymorphic) than any others previously studied. The electron microscopists who later discovered EBOV were surprised to see the crook-shaped virus particles with long tails [Ellis, 1979; Ellis 1979a; Murphy, 1978; Peters, 1969; Peters, 1971].

By comparing the differences in images when different techniques (ultrathin section and negative staining in electron microscopy) are used, it becomes apparent that some of the variety of shapes and structures are due to differences in the three-dimensional orientation of viral particles in the sample. Both negative staining and ultrathin sectioning have advantages and examination by both methods is necessary to understand how a virus is organized. Negative staining allows us to examine the surface structure and shapes of the virus, whereas the ultrathin sectioning technique enables us to see the fine details of the interior structure. Using the ultrathin sectioning techniques described in Chapter 2, examination of MARV- and ZEBOV-infected cells and animal organs demonstrates the morphological variations. These morphological variations are those that have been observed using negative staining to show individual virus shapes [Ellis, 1979; Ellis, 1979a; Geisbert, 1995; Peters, 1969; Peters, 1971].

Filoviral shapes serve as a good diagnostic feature because they differ from all other known viruses. We examined negatively stained samples of MARV and ZEBOV prepared from blood serum derived from infected guinea pigs and monkeys, and also from infected cell culture fluid. Examples of the different morphological forms of ZEBOV and MARV are presented in Figures 3-1 through 3-3. Figure 3-1 shows MARV structures in an ultrathin section. The different

Figure 3-1A

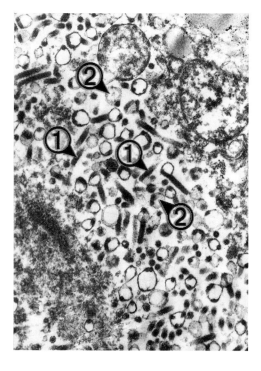

Legend

FIGURE 3-1

1. Rod-shaped

2. Polymorphous

3. 6-shaped

4. Glycoprotein (GP)

5. Viral envelope

See Note on page xiii.

Figure 3-1. Various MARV structures are visible at different magnifications in these three photos made of ultrathin sections. **Figure 3-1A** shows a section of the liver of an infected guinea pig and shows the accumulation of predominately rod-shaped and polymorphous viral particles (magnification 11,000). **Figure 3-1B** shows a 6-shaped particle and a rod-shaped particle (magnification 110,000). The striated tubular nucleocapsid, covered by the membrane envelope, is visible. The cross-striated structure of the nucleocapsid is produced by the helical packing of the ribonucleoprotein complex. **Figure 3-1C** is a cross-section of the tubular nucleocapsid of the virus (magnification 130,000). The double-layered envelope (donut-shaped) and even the surface glycoprotein (GP) can be seen forming a loop.

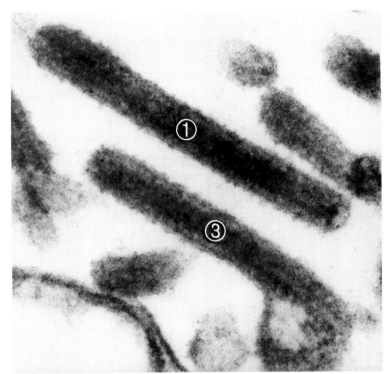

Figure 3-1B

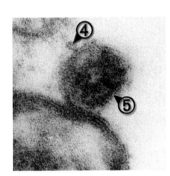

Figure 3-1C

shapes (6-shaped, ring, and rod) of MARV are apparent. Figure 3-2 also shows several different views of MARV, using a negatively stained sample of blood serum from the liver of a guinea pig. In these pictures, we see the rod-shaped, 6-shaped, branched, and ring-shaped virions.

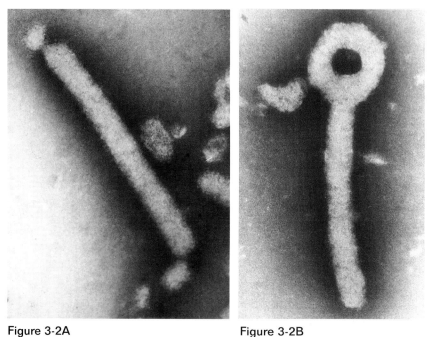

Figure 3-2A

Figure 3-2B

Figure 3-2. Various shapes of MARV virions are apparent in electron microscope pictures of negatively stained preparations (magnification 120,000). Viral suspensions were obtained from the blood of a guinea pig.
Figure 3-2A shows a rod-like MARV virion. **Figure 3-2B** shows a 6-shaped virion. **Figure 3-2C** shows branched and ring-shaped particles.

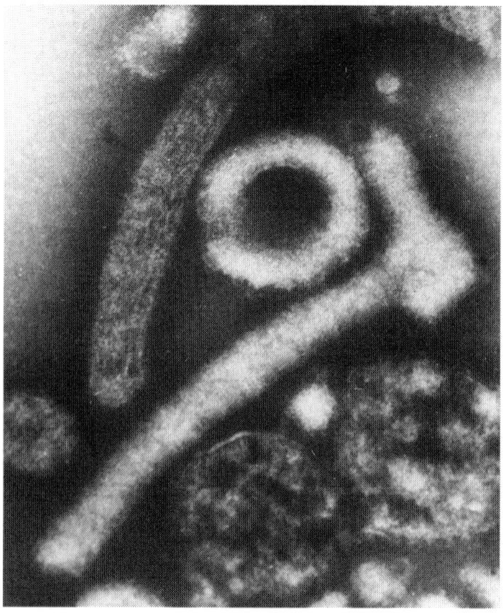

Figure 3-2C

Figure 3-3, a negatively stained image, shows several shapes of ZEBOV, including filamentous, branched, and 6-shaped particles.

General Structure of Filoviruses

The diameter of a filovirus is about 80 nm, regardless of its apparent shape, whereas its length varies widely, with the longest virions measuring up to 14 μm. MARV virions are about 790 nm in length. The MARV genome contains a single gene overlap. EBOV virions are longer, about 970 nm in length, and the genome contains several gene overlaps. Filoviral virions contain seven proteins: nucleoprotein (NP), virion structural proteins (VP24, VP30, VP35, and VP40), glycoprotein (GP), and large or polymerase protein (L). In addition, EBOV has a non-structural, small, secreted glycoprotein (sGP).

Filoviruses have a single, negative-stranded, linear RNA genome, which forms a ribonucleoprotein complex (nucleocapsid)

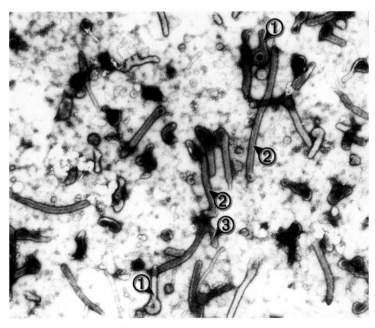

Legend

FIGURE 3-3

1. 6-shaped
2. Filamentous
3. Branched

See Note on page xiii.

Figure 3-3. Various filoviral shapes negatively stained by uranyl acetate (magnification 19,000). ZEBOV particles from the blood serum of guinea pigs (passage 7) are shown. Filamentous particles, branched particles, and 6-shaped particles are visible.

in association with nucleoprotein. The filoviral nucleocapsid is tubular, with an external diameter of 45–50 nm, and an internal diameter of approximately 19 nm when examined in ultrathin sections. The helical packing of the ribonucleoprotein complex (composed of proteins NP, L, VP35, and VP30) gives the nucleocapsid a cross-striated appearance, with an interval of about 5 nm (see the structure of MARV in Figure 3-1B). The nucleocapsid is covered by a closely adhering envelope or viral membrane. The three viral proteins associated with the membrane are GP, VP24, and VP40. The membrane envelope has projections (spikes or peplomers), visible as loops at high magnification (Figure 3-1C). The spikes are composed of GP and are not seen consistently in negatively stained preparations, especially after the virions have been subjected to sample manipulations (e.g., concentration or purification). The non-structural, small, secreted glycoprotein (sGP) of EBOV is released from the infected cell and covers the nucleocapsid [Feldmann, 1999a].

Structure and Function of Filoviral Proteins

The filoviruses' seven proteins, NP, VP35, VP40, GP, L, VP30 and VP24 give structure to the virus. The VPs and NP form the main body of the virus, and the L and VP35 form the anchor of the NP chain. The GP appears as spikes in the membrane of the nucleocapsid. Feldmann proposed the locations of the different proteins in the nucleocapsid as presented in Figure 3-4 [Feldmann, 1999]. Feldmann also summarized the proposed functions of each protein, based on analogies with other viruses (Table 3-1).

The functions of L, VPs, and NP are most closely associated with the structure and replication of the virus. The functions of GP (and sGP of EBOV) are interesting. Although GP does not appear to be the same as envelope proteins on other nonsegmented, negative strand (NNS) RNAs, there is a sequence of amino acids within the GP that is similar to a sequence in the envelope proteins of retroviruses. Moreover, this area is associated with an immunosuppressive domain in the retrovirus proteins that inhibits the transformation of small lymphocytes into larger cells capable of undergoing mitosis (blastogenesis), a decrease in monocyte chemotaxis and macrophage infiltration, and inhibition

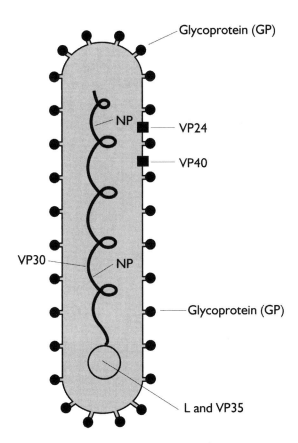

Figure 3-4. Schematic of a filovirus (adapted from Feldmann, 1999). The helical structure of the ribonucleoprotein complex is made of VP30, VP35, and NP; the L protein is at one end of the ribonucleoprotein. The capsid contains the membrane-associated proteins VP24 and VP40. The glycoprotein (GP) forms spikes or protrusions on the membrane.

Table 3-1. Proposed functions of the filoviral proteins.*

Protein	Placement	Proposed Function
NP	Ribonucleoprotein complex	Encapsidation
VP35	Ribonucleoprotein complex	Polymerase cofactor
VP40	Membrane-associated	Matrix protein
GP	Transmembrane protein	Receptor binding
sGP[†]	Non-structural, secreted	Immune modulation
VP30	Ribonucleoprotein complex	Encapsidation
VP24	Membrane-associated	Unknown (possibly a second matrix protein)
L	Ribonucleoprotein complex	RNA-dependent RNA polymerase

*Based on Feldmann (1999)
[†]EBOV only

of human natural killer (NK) cell activity. GP is the only surface protein and therefore probably plays a role in binding to cellular receptors. For these reasons, among others, GP is considered the major viral antigen and main target for the host immune response. GP is proteolytically activated by the prohormone convertase furin into two subunits GP(1) and GP(2) [Sanger, 2002]. The non-structural sGP that is secreted from EBOV-infected cells is directed into the endoplasmic reticulum of the host and is believed to modulate the host's immune response [Feldmann, 1999]. Feldmann recently published a detailed review of the properties of filoviral GPs [Feldmann, 2001].

Based on the proposed functions for GP and sGP, we can anticipate that the filoviral infections will cause diseases that disturb the immune system and, in particular, will suppress some functions. This may be more obvious in EBOV infections since the sGP may assist in affecting the immune system to a greater degree. Some of these changes may be associated with the monocytes and macrophages. For example, monocytes may not migrate towards the infection as they normally would and macrophages may not act to remove the infected cells in their normal manner. In addition, NK cells may not be stimulated to destroy and remove infected cells. While changes in these basic cellular functions may occur, modifications in the pattern of cytokines or factors released by the different cells may also occur. These modifications may induce further changes in cells not infected by the filovirus. The operation of the immune system is controlled by the responses of macrophages and lymphocytes; when these are affected, we can expect major dysfunctions of the immune system.

Infection: Penetration

The interaction of a virus and the cell surface is the heart of the infection process and may be examined by various methods. Using electron microscopy of ultrathin sections, the steps of this interaction can be directly monitored. Infection begins when a virus adsorbs on the cell and binds to a specific surface receptor by a special attachment protein(s). Virus receptors may include molecules involved in different physiological or pathological processes.

For example, the receptor for acetylcholine also serves as the receptor for the rabies virus in neural cells.

Viral particles, in general, penetrate the cell in two ways, either by using vesicles that form from the plasma membrane at the virus attachment site, or by direct fusion with the plasma membrane. The first pathway for entry is known as receptor-mediated endocytosis. Receptor-mediated endocytosis is the mode of entry for many hormones and large molecules into cells, and it is also believed to be the mechanism for such viruses as the Semliki Forest virus (a *Togavirus*) and the foot and mouth disease virus (a *Picornavirus*). When a virus uses this mechanism, it is using the natural pathway of large molecules to gain access into the cell. To enter using this method, the virus must bind to the cell surface receptors, which are concentrated in clathrin-coated pits. These pits then bud into the cell forming clathrin-coated vesicles, with the virus inside. Clathrin consists of protein chains that assemble into a basket-like structure that distorts the membrane and drives membrane budding. After the vesicle has formed and entered the cytoplasm, the viral envelope fuses with the vesicular membrane, which enables the viral nucleic acid to invade the cell cytoplasm. The schematic in Figure 3-5 illustrates the receptor-mediated endocytosis and direct fusion process. The process of receptor-mediated endocytosis is easily identified in the electron microscope by the presence of clathrin deposits on the external surface of the vesicle membrane [Barlow, 1994; Chain, 1988; Dimmock, 1982]. In the second method, direct fusion, the virus first binds to the surface receptors, then its membrane fuses with the cell envelope and the nucleocapsid emerges inside the cell, ready to replicate. This is the mechanism used by many paramyxoviruses, such as the measles virus.

The highly hazardous nature of the filoviruses has limited their experimental studies and, in general, the mode of entry of the filoviruses into the cell is unknown. After the virus binds to a receptor on the target cell, it must penetrate into the cell to release its nucleic acid into the cytoplasm and thereby trigger genome replication and viral reproduction. So far, no single receptor for the filoviruses has been identified. However, the present achievements in molecular biology have provided various model systems useful for examining the role of the molecular compounds of the filovirus

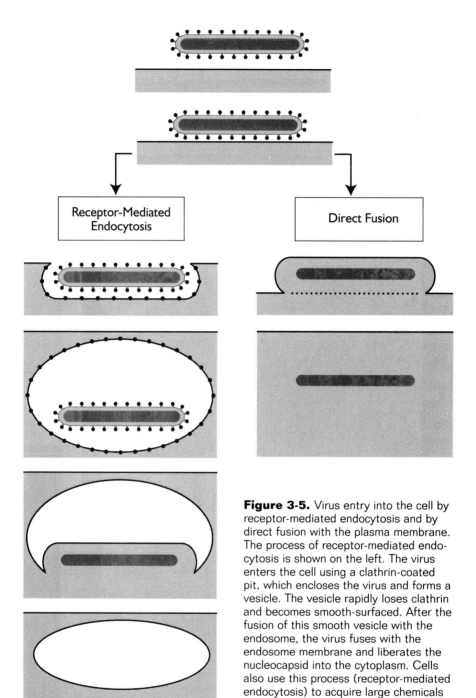

Figure 3-5. Virus entry into the cell by receptor-mediated endocytosis and by direct fusion with the plasma membrane. The process of receptor-mediated endocytosis is shown on the left. The virus enters the cell using a clathrin-coated pit, which encloses the virus and forms a vesicle. The vesicle rapidly loses clathrin and becomes smooth-surfaced. After the fusion of this smooth vesicle with the endosome, the virus fuses with the endosome membrane and liberates the nucleocapsid into the cytoplasm. Cells also use this process (receptor-mediated endocytosis) to acquire large chemicals and proteins. Direct fusion is shown on the right. Here, the virus fuses with the cell membrane and enters the cell directly without a clathrin-coated pit and without a vacuole.

during entry into cells. Using pseudotype systems, studies have found that GP of ZEBOV is the viral binding protein attaching the virus to the cellular surface [Chan, 2000; Takada, 1997; Wool-Lewis, 1998]. Chan used a pseudotype virus packaged with either MARV or ZEBOV GP to study the interaction of GP with target cells in a wide range of mammalian cells. Takada used a recombinant system based on a vesicular stomatitis virus (VSV) and EBOV GP from REBOV (the VSV was designed to express EBOV GP) to demonstrate that the GPs on the virus assist the entry of the virus into the cell but was unable to demonstrate there were any specific receptors. Filoviruses do not infect lymphocytes, as shown by Geisbert and Jaax [Geisbert, 1998; Geisbert, 2000; Jaax, 1996] and, indeed, Wool-Lewis used a pseudotyped murine leukemia virus expressing ZEBOV GP and was also unable to show that specific receptors were present on B and T lymphocyte cell membranes. Becker demonstrated that asialoglycoprotein receptors, expressed on the surface of hepatocytes, might serve as receptors (or co-receptors) for MARV in the liver [Becker, 1995]. Integrins, especially the beta 1 group, were shown to interact with the GP of EBOV, and have been proposed as receptors (or co-receptors) for EBOV [Takada, 2000]. Recent studies using artificial systems showed that both MARV and EBOV use folate receptor-alpha (FR-alpha) as a cofactor for entry into cells [Chan, 2001]. Based on the work of Takada, Chan, Becker, and Wool-Lewis, the filoviruses appear to use not just a single receptor, but a family of surface receptors to gain entry into mammalian cells.

Geisbert and Jahrling described the presence of coated vesicles in filovirus-infected cell cultures, indicating receptor-mediated endocytosis may be occurring [Geisbert, 1995]. We have also seen filoviruses associated with clathrin-coated pits in cell cultures and in sections of the visceral organs from infected animals in our studies (Figure 3-6). Figure 3-6A shows fibers between the virus and plasma membrane. For clarity, a schematic is presented in Figure 3-6B, which can guide the reader to the important details. Figure 3-6C shows no clatharin particles on the plasma membrane. However, these observations do not justify the conclusion that receptor-mediated endocytosis is the entry mode of the filoviruses into cells. In fact, the subsequent steps of endocytosis, including uncoating of the virion in the endosomes, have not been

Legend

FIGURE 3-6

1. Glycoprotein (GP)
2. Fiber
3. Clathrin particle
4. Plasma membrane

See Note on page xiii.

Figure 3-6. Patterns of receptor-mediated endocytosis of MARV; association of the virus with clathrin-coated pits. **Figure 3-6A** shows fibers visible between the virions and the cell's plasma membrane (magnification 80,000). This is morphological evidence that the virus interacts with the cellular surface. There are also clathrin particles on the outer surface of the coated pits. **Figure 3-6B** is a schematic that highlights the features in 3-6A. **Figure 3-6C** shows the clathrin coating on the cellular plasma membrane (magnification 82,000).

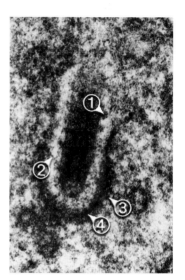

Figure 3-6A

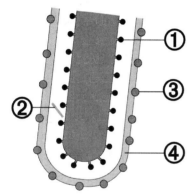

Figure 3-6B

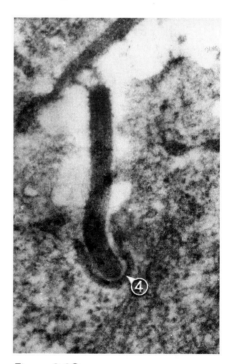

Figure 3-6C

demonstrated. It seems quite plausible that the filoviruses enter the cell mainly by fusion with the plasma membrane. Patterns confirming entry by fusion are observed in many of our cells and tissue ultrathin sections. However, these observations should also be interpreted cautiously because filoviruses budding through the plasma membrane during release from the cell produce the same morphological patterns. That is, the electron microscope pictures would appear the same whether the filoviruses are entering the cell via fusion with the plasma membrane or are budding from the membrane as they mature and leave the cell.

After analyzing the results of our observations of receptor-mediated endocytosis, we believe that MARV enters cells by this mechanism, while ZEBOV uses direct fusion with the plasma membrane. This conclusion is based on our observations of many electron micrographs of both MARV and ZEBOV. Endocytosis was common in our micrographs of MARV, whereas endocytosis was found in only one of our electron micrographs of ZEBOV. A study to directly compare the entries of MARV and ZEBOV has not been performed. However, studies using model systems showed that interactions of ZEBOV and MARV GPs with target cells were distinct, indicating they had different modes of entry into cells [Chan, 2000]. Molecular biological features of ZEBOV GP interaction with cellular membranes suggested that fusion takes place and is pH-dependent [Wool-Lewis, 1998]. More recently, studies have demonstrated that ZEBOV entry involves caveolae, which supports the view that ZEBOV entry is by endocytosis [Empig, 2002].

Clarification of the penetration pathway of the virus into the cell would certainly bring us closer to an understanding of the mechanisms underlying the development of filoviral infections and facilitate the design of drug therapies interfering with this specific phase of the viral life cycle. The penetration pathway is the first step in virus-cell interactions that has the potential to be blocked to prevent infection. Virus-specific antibodies act precisely at this step. After antibodies have bound to the surface of the virus, the virus cannot penetrate the cell. Creating neutralizing monoclonal antibodies directed to EBOV's and MARV's GP epitopes may be a promising approach for the development of effective therapeutics by preventing virus entry into cells [Hevey, 1997; Wilson, 2000]. In the future, antiviral compounds that specifically block filoviral receptors on the cell surface may be another approach to prevent filoviral infections.

Infection: Morphology of Viral Replication

Once the virus has entered the cell, the next stage is the transfer of the genomic material to the host cell's synthesizing machinery. This will allow the reproduction of viral progeny, or viral replication. It is during this replication that the virus acts as a parasite on the genetic level. The virus' genetic program causes the host cell to abandon its own functions and begin replicating the virus. Assembly of the virus, as the assembly of all supramolecular structures in living cells, develops by the binding of appropriate molecules to each other. Initially, the cell shows no apparent evidence (to the microscope) of infection—its structure (or morphology) remains unaltered. The duration of this latent period differs between viruses. For example, the latent period for the vaccinia virus is 4 hours. Using an immunocytochemical examination of cells, the first signs of MARV replication appear 11–12 hours post-inoculation [Dr. S. Becker, personal communication]. Electron microscopy studies also detect signs of infection 12 hours after MARV is applied onto monolayers.

Viral replication is associated with the appearance of new, virus-specific structures in infected cells. These structures are morphologically different from the normal cellular organelles. Taken together, the sequential changes in virus-specific structures in the infected cell and the formation of virions are known as morphogenesis. The morphology of these structures is specific for each viral family and occasionally is specific for individual viruses [Biel, 1999]. All the structures formed in the course of infection, the viral progeny among them, are referred to as morphological features of viral infection.

Many definitions are used to describe the morphological features of virus-related material present in the infected cell. Such material in the cytoplasm or cell nuclei is called "viroplasm," "viral factories," "virus-replication complexes," "inclusion bodies," or "viral inclusions." In fact, the cytoplasm and cell nucleus are the sites where viral progeny are formed from proteins and nucleic acids synthesized in the infected cell. The term "viroplasm" was introduced to designate viral material in the infected cell that was proposed to be precursor material. However, it is impossible to say definitely that the material of the "viroplasm" is used to assemble viral components. More likely, "viroplasm" represents a way to store unused molecules (i.e., those molecules remaining after viral progeny are formed). It may be more appropriate to use the terms "viral inclusion" or "inclusion body" for these areas in infected cells containing viral material because in cytology terms, "inclusion" means foreign material in a cell.

Viral inclusions in the infected cells may be seen not only with the electron microscope, but also by immunofluorescent microscopy using virus-specific antibodies labeled by chemicals visible in ultraviolet light. Using the appropriate stain, in some cases viral inclusions may be viewed with light microscopy. Immunofluorescent microscopy is widely used in laboratory practice for diagnosing and confirming infections in cell cultures. The use of immunofluorescence for structural studies using infected tissues is limited because the fluorescence gives fluorescing or bright spots (on a dark background) at the antigen locations, and these bright spots can cover the entire cell and make identification difficult. While this is not a major problem in cell cultures, it is particularly complicating in the examination of organ tissue samples.

Another way to identify infected cells is to use the immunoperoxidase technique, which is based on binding of specific antibodies with viral material in the cells. In this system, the reaction of peroxidase produces a colored substance at the binding site of the antibodies and provides the visualization. This method is very important in light microscopy studies, where there is good preservation of the tissue structure. Both infected and uninfected cells can be seen and pathological changes can be examined in the same section. Both immunofluorescent and immunoperoxidase techniques can be used to see infected cells and evaluate sizes and locations of viral inclusions. However, only electron microscopy provides the ultrastructural detail to examine the process of viral reproduction.

We examined the time course of MARV replication, hour-by-hour at 12–19 hours post-inoculation, in Vero cells. The first ultrastructural signs of MARV replication were detected 12 hours post-inoculation. Small foci of material with medium electron density, connected to the cytosolic surface of the endoplasmic reticulum (ER) and located in perinuclear areas, became apparent (see Figures 3-7 and 3-8). The structure of this material in random sections looked irregular and appeared to be composites of small grains, vesicles, and fragments of membranous tubules. These composites may be called "sponge-like" material (Figure 3-7A). Examination of sponge-like material sectioned at different planes showed the presence of helical tubules, closely adhered to each other alongside of, or immersed separately into, sponge-like material (Figure 3-7C). The viral nucleocapsids were also seen immersed in this sponge-like material. Tight adherence of helical tubules was clearly visible in cross sections of the same areas (Figure 3-7B). The inner diameter of the tubules was 17.2 ± 0.3 nm, and the outer diameter was 27.1 ± 0.5 nm. The tubules did not appear to be rigid but rather flexuous or sinuous; therefore, observations of uninterrupted longitudinal sections were rare.

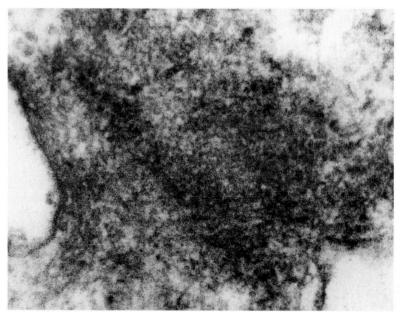

Figure 3-7A

Figure 3-7. The first evidence of MARV infection is the accumulation of viral material, which sometimes appears as a sponge-like material. **Figure 3-7A** depicts the viral inclusions in the MARV-infected Vero cells (magnification 120,000). The aggregation of sponge-like material is connected to the outer surface of the endoplasmic reticulum membrane. **Figure 3-7B** shows the cross-section of the tightly packed tubules, which may be found in the sponge-like material if we could cut a perpendicular section of the tubules (magnification 120,000). **Figure 3-7C** shows the viral nucleocapsids immersed in the sponge-like material (magnification 46,000).

Other viral structures were observed in the infected cells, in addition to sponge-like material. Studies of the expression of MARV recombinant nucleoprotein in prokaryotic and eukaryotic systems showed that the nucleoprotein formed helical tubules closely resembling the nucleocapsid in the absence of other viral proteins. Nucleoprotein has been proposed to be the main factor for determining the formation of the helical tubules, which serve as a skeleton for the MARV nucleocapsid [Kachko, 2001; Kolesnikova, 2000]. Individual helical tubules, very similar if not structurally identical to MARV nucleocapsids, were seen on the

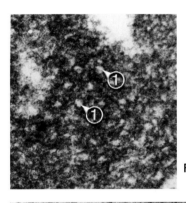

Figure 3-7B

Legend

FIGURE 3-7

1. Tubule

2. Nucleocapsid

See Note on page xiii.

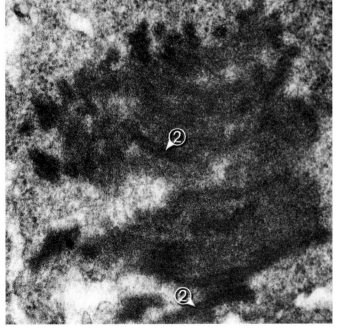

Figure 3-7C

Legend

FIGURE 3-8

1. Nucleocapsid

2. Endoplasmic
   reticulum (ER)
   membrane

3. Lucent vesicle

See Note on page xiii.

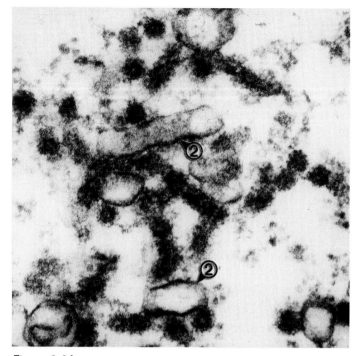

Figure 3-8A

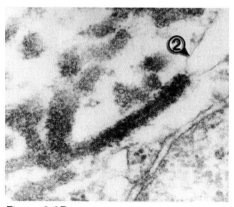

Figure 3-8B

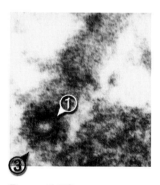

Figure 3-8C

Figure 3-8. Various sections showing the formation and appearance of MARV nucleocapsids. **Figure 3-8A** shows the development of sheets and chains of nucleocapsids connected with the surface of the endoplasmic reticulum (ER) (magnification 58,000). The nucleocapsids have a villous surface (they look like hairy caterpillars). These nucleocapsids are sectioned at various planes, so not all of them show the distinct central tubular hole. **Figure 3-8B** shows the connection of nucleocapsids with the ER surface (magnification 55,000). **Figure 3-8C** shows the small lucent vesicle that crowns each protrusion on the nucleocapsid, as well as details of the protrusions on the nucleocapsid surface (magnification 120,000).

outer surface of ER (Figure 3-8A) in infected cells, indicating that
the helices may be capable of self-assembly. For clarity, we called
these tubules connected with the ER "primary nucleocapsids,"
while the term "nucleocapsid" was reserved for those unassociated
nucleocapsids in the cytoplasm outside of the inclusion areas.
Primary nucleocapsids were connected with the ER by their lateral
surface or by their end (Figures 3-8A and 3-8B). They had an outer
diameter of 53 ± 0.4 nm. Primary nucleocapsids looked villous at
low magnification, while at high magnification, small, electron-
dense protrusions were apparent on their outer surface. A small
lucent vesicle seemed to crown each protrusion (Figure 3-8C).
These same structures were observed on the surface of nucleocapsids of complete virions. We compared the primary nucleocapsids
with nucleocapsids of complete viral particles and with nucleocapsids prepared for budding. The primary nucleocapsids differed
in appearance from both of these only by having slightly less
electron density and a slightly less clear-cut appearance.

The viral structures involved in the formation of MARV
inclusions are shown in a schematic (Figure 3-9). Studies of serial
sections of the infected cell showed that both primary nucleocapsids
and conglomerates of material with a sponge-like appearance may

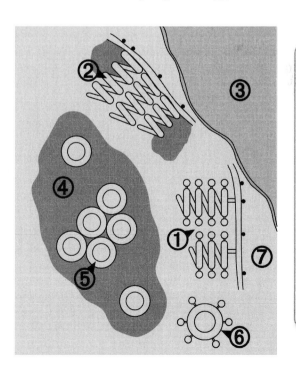

Figure 3-9.
Schematic of
formation of MARV
inclusions. The
inclusions represent
a composite of
spongy material,
dense tubular
conglomerates,
and separate
nucleocapsids.

Legend

Figure 3-9

1. Nucleocapsid
2. Tightly packed
   tubule
3. Nucleus of
   infected cell
4. Sponge-like
   material
5. Cross-section of
   dense tubular
   conglomerate
6. Cross-section of
   nucleocapsid
7. Endoplasmic
   reticulum (ER)

See Note on page xiii.

be connected with different ER profiles inside one cell. In addition, several foci of the viral material may be seen at one of the ER membranes. The developing structures approach each other and interlace, thereby creating an incredibly diversified, complex structure. It appears that the growing viral material occupies more and more space in the cytoplasm, displaces the cellular organelles, and forms a viral inclusion. Taken together, all viral structures growing in the same cell generate a unique three-dimensional picture, which provides the characteristic images of MARV-infected cells. Electron microscopic examination of serial sections of different cells showed that all the structural diversities of MARV inclusion bodies were a result of the random collocation of nucleocapsids, chains and palisades composed of nucleocapsids, sponge-like material, and tightly packed tubules. Two of the typical structural varieties of MARV inclusion bodies are shown in Figure 3-10.

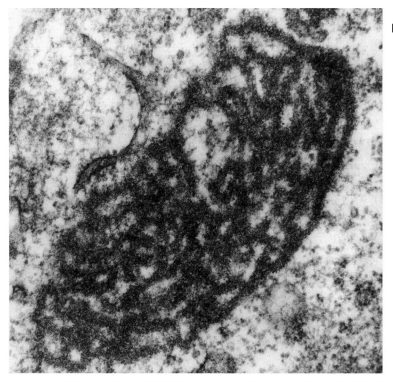

Figure 3-10A

Figure 3-10. MARV inclusions in Vero cells. **Figure 3-10A** shows inclusions composed of mostly sheets and chains of nucleocapsids (magnification 32,000). The inclusion shown in **Figure 3-10B** is composed of sponge-like material, with tightly packed nucleocapsids (magnification 34,000).

Unfortunately, we did not have the opportunity to perform an hour-by-hour examination of ZEBOV replication. We examined ZEBOV replication in Vero and L-68 cells at 24, 48, and 72 hours post-inoculation. We compared the sections of ZEBOV- and MARV-infected cells for different patterns of nucleocapsid assembly. The nucleocapsids in ZEBOV-infected cells appeared straight and separated from each other by fine granular material (Figure 3-11). Since the nucleocapsids generally were parallel, the inclusion bodies usually had rectangular shapes. A chaotic arrangement of ZEBOV nucleocapsids was rare, and so inclusion bodies rarely showed shapes that may be described as odd or irregular. In fact, when ZEBOV inclusions were irregular, the virions did not appear to have nucleocapsids. For comparison with MARV inclusions, look at Figure 3-8, where MARV nucleocapsids were connected to the ER surface and each other in chains and sheets.

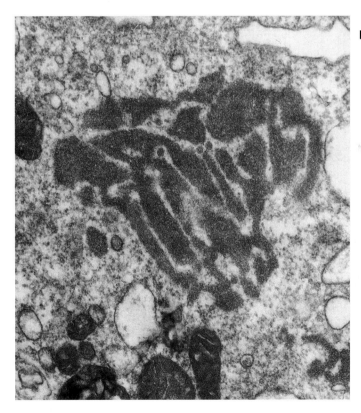

Figure 3-10B

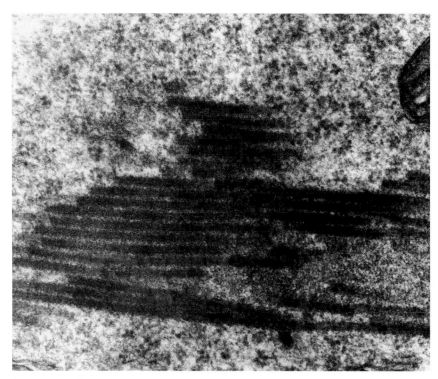

Figure 3-11A

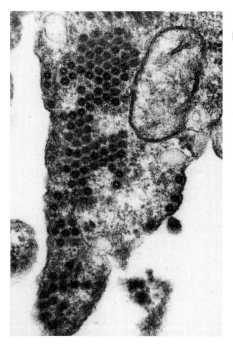

Figure 3-11B

Figure 3-11. Nucleocapsids of ZEBOV in longitudinal and cross-sectional views. **Figure 3-11A** shows a longitudinal view where each nucleocapsid is separate, but the groupings are regular (magnification 80,000). **Figure 3-11B** is a cross-sectional view of the nucleocapsid (magnification 78,000).

The images of inclusion bodies produced by MARV and ZEBOV cannot be confused and the difference serves as a diagnostic tool for the two filoviruses.

Occasionally there were helices apparent in the cytoplasm of ZEBOV-infected cells; however, few nucleocapsids were found among these helices (Figure 3-12). This type of pattern was rarely observed in MARV-infected cells. Images showing helices were found in the cells of organs in infected animals but were not detected in cell cultures. We believe that these structures (helices) result from a replication process that has been interrupted due to insufficient cell synthetic capacities.

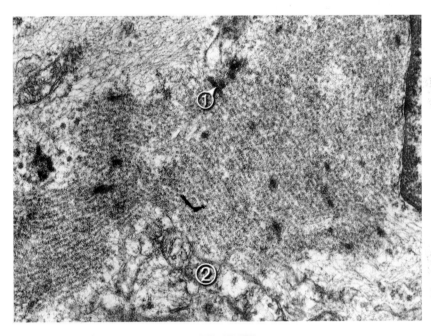

Legend

Figure 3-12

1. Nucleocapsid
2. Mitochondria

See Note on page xiii.

Figure 3-12A

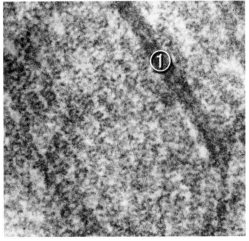

Figure 3-12. ZEBOV inclusion composed of helices. **Figure 3-12A** shows the few nucleocapsids that are found among the collection of coiled tubules (magnification 21,500). This is evidence that the normal replication has been disrupted because such structures (tubules) are not usually seen in cells. With this many nucleoproteins in the cell, we would expect to see that many more nucleocapsids have formed. Mitochondria can also be seen. **Figure 3-12B** also shows a nucleocapsid and helices (magnification 100,000).

Figure 3-12B

Infection: Viral Budding

As with many enveloped viruses, filoviruses acquire their outer envelope by passing through the cellular membrane and covering the genome with these membranes. This process is called "budding" and is really two steps: 1) the enveloping of the nucleocapsid, and 2) the exiting of the virion from the host cell. As the first step in budding, the nucleocapsid approaches the internal surface of the plasma membrane. Next, the nucleocapsid bulges outward and is covered by the membrane. In the last step of budding, the enveloped virion detaches from the surface. Both MARV and EBOV are enveloped viruses and follow the same steps in budding.

In our EM studies of MARV, we were able to obtain a detailed view and document the steps in MARV budding. MARV budding is presented in Figures 3-13 through 3-16. Figure 3-17 is a schematic that aids in the visualization of these steps. Although the viral membrane must close when the virion leaves the cell, this particular step has not been observed with the EM. In our studies, we noticed that small "bubbles" seem to link the virion with the cell surface. These bubbles can be seen in Figures 3-14C and 3-14D. These bubbles may represent the very last step of enveloping as the virion leaves the cell.

The shape of the budding determines the shapes of the viral particles. Rod-shaped virions can be formed by the movement of the nucleocapsid either parallel or perpendicular to the cell membrane. In the case of parallel budding, the membrane simultaneously covers the nucleocapsid along the whole length of the viral particle. The virion then moves forward evenly along its entire length and emerges from the cell. The nucleocapsid can also contact the membrane perpendicularly or at other angles, causing one end of the nucleocapsid to contact the cell membrane and push through the cell membrane as a finger pushes through a balloon or rubber membrane. The ring-shaped and 6-shaped virions also form during budding. Soon after ring-shaped virions were first observed, researchers suggested that the ring variants were formed from nucleocapsids that were liberated from the cells during the cell destruction and were formed outside the cells during a maturation process [Almeida, 1971]. Ellis assumed that the ring variants could be formed on the ends of the long EBOV particles or by closure of the short virions [Ellis, 1978a]. Our studies have shown that ring-shaped particles appear when budding starts from the central part of nucleocapsid, as it lies parallel to the plasma membrane, while the ends of the nucleocapsid lag. The budding virion looks similar to the handle of suitcase. A disk, which is very thin in the center, is formed, and the nucleocapsid lies at its periphery. On ultrathin cross-sections, such virions have distinct outer membranes but their inner membranes are not visible. These disks become ring particles as their central membranes are disrupted. The different budding patterns, and even the bubble on the existing virions, appear to be a result of the differences in how the nucleocapsid is bound to the cell membrane.

An examination of ultrathin sections of filovirus-infected cells shows that all the diverse morphological shapes (rings, rods, club-shaped, and filaments) are present during filoviral budding. Figure 3-13 shows a MARV nucleocapsid contacting the membrane via the vesicles on top of its protrusions. Figure 3-14 shows

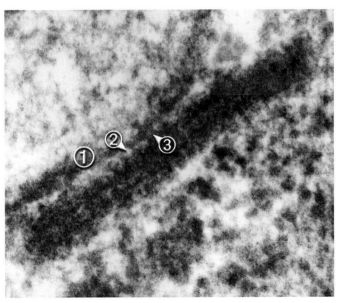

Legend

FIGURE 3-13

1. Plasma membrane
2. Small vesicle crown
3. Contact of nucleocapsid protrusions with cell membrane

See Note on page xiii.

Figure 3-13. MARV budding (magnification 116,000). The beginnings of the budding of MARV nucleocapsid and the nucleocapsid's fine structure are shown. A very distinct protrusion, crowned by a small vesicle on the nucleocapsid's outer surface, can be seen. This protrusion is approaching the cell membrane, while the adjacent protrusions are in contact with the cell membrane.

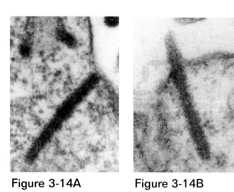

Figure 3-14A   Figure 3-14B

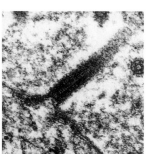

Figure 3-14C

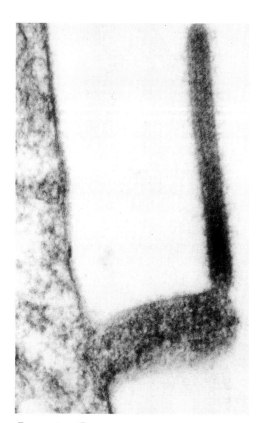

Figure 3-14D

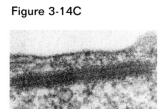

Figure 3-14E

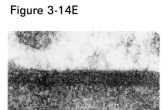

Figure 3-14F

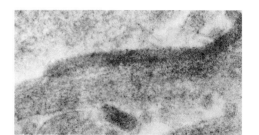

Figure 3-14G

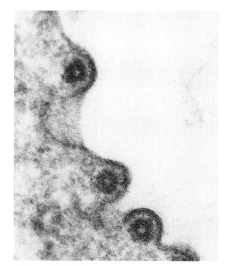

Figure 3-14H

◀ **Figure 3-14.** Different patterns of the beginning stages of MARV budding. In **Figure 3-14A** (magnification 92,000), the MARV nucleocapsid moves out towards the cell membrane, and in **Figure 3-14B** (magnification 78,000), the bud is beginning to form. **Figures 3-14C** (magnification 80,000) and **3-14D** (magnification 87,500) show the last steps in the budding. **Figures 3-14E** (magnification 45,000), **3-14F** (magnification 54,000), and **3-14G** (magnification 60,000) show the same process, but in this case, the nucleocapsid lines up alongside the membrane and the rod-shaped virion also forms. **Figure 3-14H** is a high magnification of one of the same steps in the budding of ZEBOV (magnification 146,000).

different patterns of the beginning stages of MARV budding, including the sequential steps of budding that produce rod-shaped viral particles (one of these steps is also shown for the budding of ZEBOV). Figure 3-15 shows variations in budding that lead to ring-shaped virions for MARV. The "suitcase handle" budding shape can be seen in Figure 3-15A and is the beginning of the formation of ring-shaped virions. Ring-shaped virions were commonly detected in MARV preparations but were rarely seen in ZEBOV preparations.

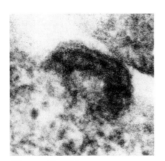

Figure 3-15A

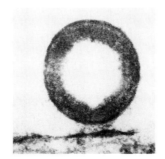

Figure 3-15B

Figure 3-15. Variations in budding that lead to ring-shaped virions for MARV. In **Figure 3-15A**, the nucleocapsid moves towards the cell membrane longitudinally, but at the beginning of the budding, the two ends of the nucleocapsid lag behind the center portion and create a "suitcase handle" shape (magnification 102,000). In **Figure 3-15B**, the virion has emerged as a ring; the lagging ends of the MARV nucleocapsid are the last part to leave the cell and have merged (magnification 105,000).

A freeze-etching picture of a MARV suspension in Figure 3-16 clearly shows rod and disc-shaped virions. For clarification, we have drawn the budding process schematically (Figure 3-17). By comparing the stages of budding shown in the schematic in Figure 3-17 with Figures 3-14 and 3-15, the process becomes clearer. Figure 3-18 shows budding of ZEBOV in an infected chick embryo cell and also shows all the stages of viral replication (i.e., viral inclusion, movement of the nucleocapsids to the cell membrane, and viral budding).

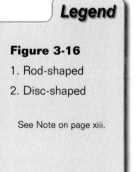

Legend

Figure 3-16

1. Rod-shaped

2. Disc-shaped

See Note on page xiii.

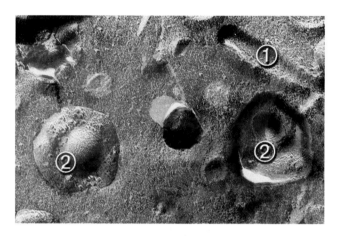

Figure 3-16. A freeze-etching picture of a MARV suspension clearly showing rod- and disc-shaped virions (magnification 80,000). (Photo by Dr. B. Zaitsev)

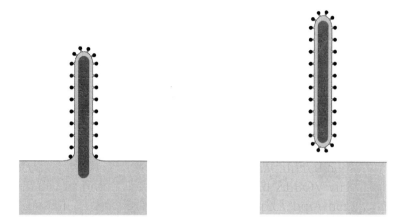

A. Perpendicular budding of rod-shaped particles.

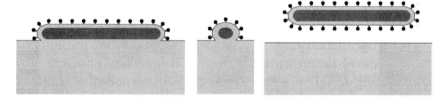

B. Longitudinal budding of rod-shaped particles (center view is a cross-section).

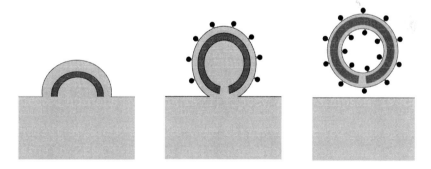

C. Budding of ring-shaped particles.

Figure 3-17. Schematic of the viral budding process for filoviruses. The budding process determines the shape of the virion particles. Compare this schematic with the EM photographs in Figures 3-14 and 3-15. The process shown in **Figure 3-17A** corresponds to Figures 3-14A, 3-14B, 3-14C, and 3-14D. The process in **Figure 3-17B** is that seen in Figures 3-14E, 3-14F, 3-14G, and 3-14H. **Figure 3-17C** is the schematic corresponding to the process in Figure 3-15 that leads to ring-shaped virions.

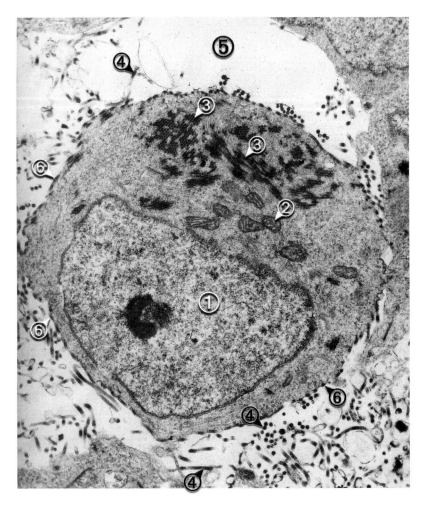

Figure 3-18. ZEBOV-infected cell of chick embryo (magnification 10,700). The entire surface of the cell shows extensive virion budding. Viral progeny particles can be seen in the intercellular space.

The way in which the nucleocapsid binds to the cell membranes results from variations in the relative positions occupied by the viral components that are responsible for binding the nucleocapsid and plasma membrane. This in turn produces the small bubbles on the virion and the irregular-shaped virions. The bubbles on the virion surface and the irregularity of club-shaped virions may be visualized as a zipper with missing teeth or as a zipper with teeth interlocked in one groove. The bubbles appear in the regions where there is too much plasma membrane (i.e., where, using the zipper image, the membrane bunches up). In contrast, when there is not enough plasma membrane, the nucleocapsid bends to accommodate itself into the preformed membrane and, in such a case, the particles become club-shaped or 6-shaped. If the envelope covers several nucleocapsids, the particles appear branched. Although the specific molecular components responsible for filoviral budding have not been determined, different budding patterns may be caused by changes in the relative positions of GP and VP40 when the nucleocapsid is binding to plasma membrane. However, Sanger showed that the GP of MARV was not a critical factor for budding [Sanger, 2001]. The main factor responsible for MARV budding is probably VP40 (analogous to the matrix protein in rhabdoviruses such as rabies, and paramyxoviruses such as measles and mumps). Recent studies showed VP40 was present at the sites of MARV budding in primary macrophages [Kolesnikova, 2002].

The viral replication and budding cycles do change over the course of filoviral infections. Our studies showed that MARV particles began to appear 20–21 hours post-inoculation in Vero cells and that the virions were actively budding for 36 hours, after which the budding patterns became scarce. The duration of the replication cycle of ZEBOV has not yet been determined; however, elements of the replication have been described elsewhere [Feldmann, 1999]. During the active budding period, the number of rod-shaped virions decreased, while the quantity of polymorphous and aberrant virions grew. At 21–26 hours post-inoculation, approximately 85–90% of the released MARV particles were rod-shaped. After 28 hours post-inoculation, the number of ring-shaped, branched, and various bubble-shaped particles increased considerably until at 72 hours, about 35–40% of the particles were not rod-shaped.

Are virions of different shapes functionally equal? Are rod-shaped virions as infective as those of ring-shaped, 6-shaped, and branched forms? Are their other properties the same? Regretfully, so far there has been no way to separate filoviral virions according to their shapes. Our studies demonstrated that rod-shaped virions are formed both in cell cultures and infected animals early during infection. The number of rod-shaped virions in the blood of filovirus-infected monkeys decreased over the course of the infection, while the number of 6-shaped, branched, and ring forms increased. As part of the time course study of the infections of monkeys with MARV, we calculated the number of virions in blood samples. The blood samples were obtained daily. On day 4 post-inoculation, 86% of the virions were rod-shaped, but by day 8, only 54% of the virions were rod-shaped. Because of their dominance, it is reasonable to suppose that rod-shaped virions represent "normal" particles, but it is impossible to say anything about how "normal" the other morphological varieties are.

Sometimes the filoviral budding process generates very unusual membranous structures. The ZEBOV reproduction process generates remarkable net-like (or cancellous) formations, which are derived from plasma membrane, at the viral budding sites (Figure 3-19). The meshes of these peculiar spheres have wavy contours. Viral particles can be seen within and around the meshes. We succeeded in following the steps in the formation of these spherical, net-like structures. We found that the structures are related to the sites of defective particle budding (Figure 3-19A). The budding particles fuse with the formation of folds, which droop on the cell surface, and acquire a membrane with a net-like appearance. We also observed defective viral particles between membrane folds (Figure 3-19B). The net-like structures are possible evidence of the cell's inability to produce viral proteins in the amounts needed for complete virion formation.

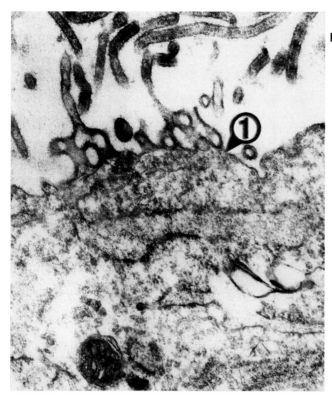

Figure 3-19A

Figure 3-19. The development of net-like structures in filovirus-infected cells.
Figure 3-19A shows the initial stages of net-like structures forming in ZEBOV infection (magnification 39,000). The cellular plasma membrane, folds made by the budding of defective virions, and defective ZEBOV particles can be seen.
Figure 3-19B shows well-developed foldings between two cells and defective ZEBOV particles (magnification 30,000). **Figure 3-19C** (page 52) shows a net-like sphere in a ZEBOV-infected cell (magnification 25,000). Regular meshes are visible and such structures are regular in visceral organs of ZEBOV-infected animals. **Figure 3-19D** (page 52) shows folds resembling net-like structures in MARV-infected cells (magnification 32,000).

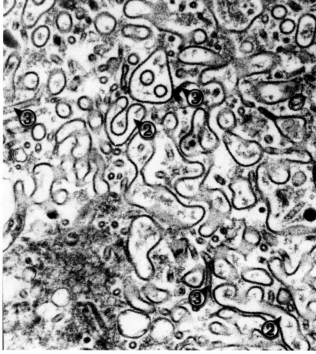

Figure 3-19B

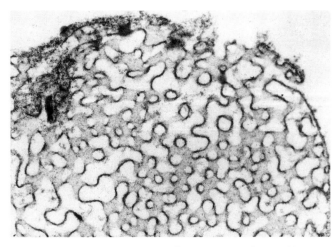

Figure 3-19C

Figure 3-19. . . . Figure 3-19C shows part of a net-like sphere in a ZEBOV-infected cell (magnification 25,000). Regular meshes are visible and such structures are regular in visceral organs of ZEBOV-infected animals.

Legend

FIGURE 3-19

1. Plasma membrane

2. Well-developed folding

3. Defective viral particle

4. Viral particle

See Note on page xiii.

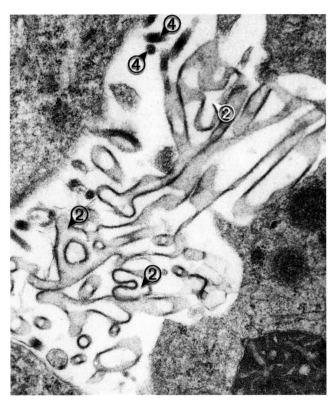

Figure 3-19D

Figure 3-19. . . . Figure 3-19D shows folds resembling net-like structures in MARV-infected cells (magnification 32,000).

Net-like spheres (Figure 3-19C) were common in the organs of ZEBOV-infected animals, while cell cultures either exhibited signs of the spheres or showed rare foldings. Net-like structures were comparatively rare in MARV infection and spheres usually were not found. Only stray folds were encountered on the plasma membrane in MARV-infected cells and animals (Figure 3-19D).

MARV and ZEBOV bud in Vero cell cultures, both on protrusions and depressions of the cells' surface areas. The entire cell surface can be involved in virion formation, and in such instances, the surface bristles with budding viral particles (Figure 3-19A). Differentiated cells have specific functions for different parts of their plasma membrane and enveloped viruses commonly have associations with specific parts of the plasma membrane in these polarized cells. Our studies showed that in polarized Madin-Darby canine kidney (MDCK) cell cultures, MARV budding occurred only on the basolateral plasma membranes, in contrast to non-polarized Vero cells [Sanger, 2001]. The same pattern was observed in infected animals: non-polarized macrophages and fibroblasts produced MARV particles on the entire surface, while budding in polarized hepatocytes was strongly restricted to the basolateral surface. This budding restriction probably is related to differences in the properties of polarized epithelial cells.

Our hour-by-hour examination of MARV-infected cells showed how complex the virus reproduction step is and how difficult that step is to study. Indeed, when a sample was examined at 48 hours post-inoculation, there was a mixture of the cells that had stopped new virus production and those that were actively producing the virus (secondary infection). These active cells differ in their metabolism and viral synthesis. This should be taken in account when molecular events of the viral infection are examined. Examining cells at synchronous stages of infection is the only way to obtain reliable data about the intrinsic mechanisms of virus-cell interaction.

Conclusion

MARV and ZEBOV reproduction is characterized by the formation of cytoplasmic inclusion bodies. The cytoplasmic inclusion bodies and their peculiarities are unique to each virus. Filoviral infections

produce polymorphous viral particles, which are formed by budding on the cell surface. We described the common features of
ZEBOV and MARV replication, but we also noted the most
frequently found structural abnormalities in filoviral infection. We
have summarized our findings in Table 3-2.

We described a pattern of the morphogenesis of MARV (strain
Popp) and ZEBOV in a cell culture system. The cells in the continuous laboratory cultures had very similar morphologic and
metabolic parameters, so they provided identical conditions for
viral reproduction. As expected, the morphological patterns of
viral reproduction were very similar in these cells. However, in
filovirus-infected animals, there were varied morphological patterns, even in the same types of infected cells. This pattern diver-
sity was related to the asynchronous infection of the cells and to
the presence of different generations of infected cells in the animal
organs. Many variants of aberrant structures may be found in the
organs of filovirus-infected animals. However, all these variants
may be evaluated using the morphological pattern of a single viral
replication cycle described above. Using these descriptions, we can
analyze viral reproduction in filovirus-infected animals and follow
the pathological changes in the visceral organs.

In addition, our hour-by-hour examination of MARV infection
and replications in Vero cells indicates that the duration of the
replication cycle is about 21 hours. Not only that, but after 28
hours, the number of normal or rod-shaped virions decreased and
the number of aberrant virions (ring, club, branched, and 6-shaped
virions) increased, suggesting that the cell has run out of the material needed to reliably replicate the filoviruses. In later chapters,
we will discuss the fact that these altered or aberrant forms of the
virus may not function in the same manner as the regular or rod-
shaped virions.

Table 3-2. Summary of differences in morphological characteristics for MARV (strain Popp) and ZEBOV infections.

Characteristic	MARV (strain Popp)	ZEBOV
Viral inclusion body	Irregular shape. Sponge-like material, random locations of nucleocapsids, helical tubules, chains and sheets.	Rectangular shape. Nucleocapsids are straight, parallel, and separated in a regular pattern.
Viral budding	Rod shapes early; rings, clubs, branches, 6-shapes later in infection. Replication cycle about 21 hours.	Rod or filamentous, club, crook and branched shapes. Ring shapes rare. Net-like structures at budding sites. Replication cycle unknown.
Viral particles	First seen 21 hours post-inoculation, Vero cells.	Within 36 hours for guinea pigs.

chapter 4

Filoviral Infections

It is very important to understand how filoviruses invade animals and humans in order to develop effective treatment and prophylaxis regimes. The mechanism by which filoviruses emerge from nature and infect the primary case is not known. But we do know how the filoviruses are transmitted between humans. Both aspects are important in preventing or mitigating the effects of filoviral outbreaks. It is important to identify the virus' target cells and subsequent steps in the progress of the infection in order to control the spread of viruses. If we know the target cells, we can begin to understand the mechanisms as the infection develops. Consequently, we can develop approaches to arrest the infection early in the disease. The evidence that a cell is the target cell must include not just the presence of the virus in the cell, but must show that the cell efficiently supports viral replication.

Filoviral Reservoirs

The reservoirs that are the natural hosts of filoviruses have not yet been identified. To be an effective natural host or virus carrier, the natural host must survive the infection long enough to support the

replication of the virus and to introduce the virus into a susceptible population. The reservoir of a filovirus acts as the mechanism that ensures survival of the filoviruses in nature. The
various monkey species that have been used in laboratory
experiments cannot be the natural hosts for the filoviruses
because the monkeys usually die within 3–16 days after inoculation. Therefore, the virus cannot survive.

There have been several attempts to identify the possible natural hosts and carriers of EBOV. During the summer of 1995,
following an outbreak of Ebola fever, an attempt was made to find
EBOV in vertebrates and arthropods collected in Zaire. Teams of
researchers from the US Centers for Disease Control and Prevention (CDC) and the US Army Medical Research Institute of Infectious Diseases (USAMRIID), operating under the umbrella of the
World Health Organization (WHO), collected and processed large
numbers of specimens, but filoviruses were not detected in any
sample. In 1995–96 Dr. R. Swanepoel and his colleagues from
South Africa tried a different approach. They injected ZEBOV
(Zaire strain) into various vertebrates, invertebrates, and even
plants and then looked for evidence of ZEBOV replication in these
species. They examined 33 varieties of 24 plant species (weeds and
crop plants) and 19 vertebrate and invertebrate species (including
pigeons, snakes, cockroaches, frogs, toads, tortoises, spiders,
snails, mice, and bats). With the exception of a few controls, such
as NIH mice and cockroaches from the Bureau of Standards in
Praetoria, the animal species were collected from Kruger National
Park in South Africa. ZEBOV replicated only in bats. Three species
of bats were used (*Tadarida condylura*, *T. pumila*, and *Epom-
phorus wahlergi*). Titers of ZEBOV from $10^{4.6}$ to $10^{7.0}$ PFU/mL
were measured in lung tissue of the bats, and titers of $10^{2.0}$ to
$10^{6.5}$ PFU/mL were measured in the pooled viscera of fruit bats.
The feces of one fruit bat also contained ZEBOV. Antigen positive
cells were detected in the lungs of an insectivorous bat by
immunohistochemistry. No evidence of viral replication was
found in the other species [Swanepoel, 1996]. According to several
reports of the outbreaks, some index patients had contact with
bats or their excretions. Thus, it is plausible that bats may be a
natural host for filoviruses.

In 1997, another attempt was made to find the filovirus' natural host in the Central African Republic. Organs of 242 common small terrestrial mammals living in peripheral forest areas were examined for the presence of EBOV. Sequences of EBOV GP or polymerase genes were detected by reverse transcription PCR in RNA extracts of seven animals, and by PCR in the DNA extract of one animal. The animals belonged to two genera of rodents (*Muridae, Mus setulosus; Muridae, Praomys* sp1 and sp2) and one belonged to a shrew species (*Soricidae, Sylvisorex ollula*). The virus sequences were identified as being related to ZEBOV (strain Gabon). These data are very interesting and promising, but the investigators did not find an isolate virus or even detect viral antigens in any of the samples obtained from those seven animals [Morvan, 1999].

Swanepoel's approach to infecting animals and plants to find those species in which the virus replicates is more likely to be successful than examining hundreds of samples in the hopes that one sample might contain the virus. However, his results indicate only that the virus can replicate in bats. There is no conclusive evidence that they are the natural hosts or reservoirs for the virus. In fact, bats have been implicated as hosts in several other viruses, including Nipah virus, a paramyxovirus. Nipah virus isolates have been found in bat feces and urine in Malaysia, which along with serological evidence identified two species of bats as natural reservoirs of the virus [Chua, 2002]. If a filovirus can be isolated from bats in their natural environment, it will confirm that bats are natural hosts. Since there are large numbers of bats, and only rare outbreaks of filoviral hemorrhagic fever, only a few bats may be needed as hosts. The task of finding these few infected bats is very difficult, and it is not surprising that the attempts to find infected hosts were unsuccessful.

A very interesting hypothesis regarding the natural cycle of EBOV has been proposed, based on ecological studies of free-living chimpanzees in the Tai National Park of the Ivory Coast. The mortality of apes has been monitored since 1979, and these data were used in an epidemiological investigation of an Ebola fever outbreak in 1994. Dead Colobus monkeys were found during this outbreak and it was noted that chimpanzees that fed on Colobus monkeys were five times more likely to be infected with CIEBOV.

Based on these data, the following model was proposed. Chimpanzees regularly hunt monkeys, and the Western Red Colobus (*Colobus badius badius*) is their predominant prey. An investigation of the apes' mortality showed that Colobus could have been the source of CIEBOV infection of apes, and the Colobus might be an intermediate host (i.e., a host that is itself contaminated periodically by the true reservoir). Colobus monkeys could be contaminated from food, from specific arthropods of the upper strata of the forest, or through contact with excretions from rodents, bats, or other vertebrates. It is possible that studies of Colobus ecology could identify which species could be the candidate reservoir [Formenty, 1999a].

Transmission Between Humans

The problem of filoviral spread among humans has been investigated but the details of the mechanisms for transmission are not understood. Retrospective epidemiological studies revealed that people might be infected with MARV and EBOV through blood or secretions of patients or animals, and through traces of blood in syringes and needles in hospitals. The recent outbreak of ZEBOV infections in Gabon was arrested by quarantine, barrier nursing, and other medical care measures [WHO, 1996]. But when medical care or quarantine measures have not been vigorously pursued, the outbreaks have been difficult to contain and arrest [WHO, 2002].

Although the ways in which filoviruses emerge from nature and spread among humans are important at the population level, the problem of the filoviral infection of a single individual is also important. For example, in one report, there were 300 contacts with a person who was sick with Ebola fever and only one of the contacts displayed any sign of the infection. The contact died, but the source patient survived [Richards, 2000]. The severity of the disease depends at least in part on the mode of transmission, and obviously, not all of the transmission modes have been determined. The severity of the disease also depends on various individual host response factors. The most severe forms of filoviral disease developed in humans who were exposed via sharps and needles (i.e., when the filovirus was administered directly into the bloodstream). However, reports of the epidemiological studies are occasionally puzzling and can contain conflicting or insufficient information. For example, transmission rates cannot be determined when it is not clear how many contacts of symptomatic patients actually contract the disease. If the report says EBOV was transmitted by an unknown fashion among a group of patients who survived the infection, how can transmission and mortality rates be calculated? In another study, EBOV was also reported as transmitted in an unknown manner, with some of the patients showing no clinical symptoms of Ebola fever, yet their blood contained evidence of the virus. These patients received no therapy and care in hospitals and could not have become infected by syringes and needles contaminated by infectious blood [LeRoy, 2000].

Experimental Studies of Filoviral Infection

There are few published studies describing experimental filoviral infections and most of these have been performed with very high doses of virus. Early filoviral studies established experimentally that susceptible animals could be infected by various routes (subcutaneous, intramuscular, intravenous, aerosol, intracerebral, or conjunctival routes) using infected cell culture fluids, organ suspensions, or blood samples from filovirus-infected subjects [Haas, 1971; Peters, 1991; Siegert, 1972]. Aerosol transmission is considered an important route for the transmission of the filoviruses. Several experimental studies, using special chambers and aerosol generators, have shown that monkeys and guinea pigs may be infected by the aerosol route [Johnson, 1995; Lub, 1995; Pyankov, 1995]. However, these experiments do not provide any insight into the efficiency of aerosols in natural transmission because the animals were exposed to very high doses of the virus.

Transmission Mode and Disease

Development of viremia (presence of virus in the blood) is important to the filoviral disease's progression and transmission. Viremia means a generalized infection and is the critical step in the disease progression. While suspected, the inoculation route and dose were not proven to influence the time period for the filovirus' entry into the bloodstream. We can use our experiments to address these aspects, which are summarized in Table 4-1. When the dose given was relatively small, the time to detection of virus in the blood increased. Following an aerosol exposure of 10^5 LD_{50}, MARV was detected in the blood of guinea pigs in only 2 hours; however, following a dose of 2–5 LD_{50} the filovirus was detected only after 72 hours [Ryabchikova, 1996a]. MARV injected intraperitoneally in guinea pigs and green monkeys at a dose of 100 LD_{50} (for guinea pigs) was also found in the blood 24 hours

Table 4-1. The relation between dose and inoculation mode on the time of filoviral detection in blood (viremia).*

Virus	Infectious Dose	Inoculation Mode	Animals	Time to Viremia	Method of Detection	Reference
MARV	10^5 LD_{50}	Aerosol	Guinea pigs	2 h	Guinea pig inoculation	Ryabchikova, 1996a
EBOV	10^5 PFU	Subcutaneous injection	Rhesus monkeys	24 h	PFU in Vero cells	Fischer-Hoch, 1985
MARV	10^2 LD_{50}	Intraperitoneal injection	Green monkeys/ Guinea pigs	24 h	Guinea pig inoculation	Ryabchikova, 1994
ZEBOV	5 LD_{50}	Aerosol	Rhesus moneys	72 h	PFU in Vero cells	Pyankov, 1995
MARV	2–5 LD_{50}	Aerosol	Guinea pigs	72 h	Guinea pig inoculation	Ryabchikova, 1996a
ZEBOV	20 LD_{50}	Subcutaneous injection	Baboons	4 days	Innoculation of newborn mice	Luchko, 1995
				5 days	PFU in Vero cells	

Special Note: Examination of viremia using animal or cell culture systems is a routine examination in virology studies. However, the sensitivity of such assays to measure the total viral burden is frequently unknown. Indeed, only a small amount of blood is used for the examination (about 1 mL from monkeys). It is easy to imagine that after the virus replicates in the primary infected cells and the virions are released, not all of the virions immediately reach the bloodstream, particularly if the primary infected cell is outside of the circulatory system. The newly formed virions may infect contiguous cells and produce an additional replication cycle before they reach the blood. Despite this, the filoviruses appear in the blood quite rapidly, even at low infecting doses. Viremia also depends on the detectability of the viruses in the blood. In the case of filoviral infections, the concentration of virus in the blood must be sufficient to detect by routine biotitration. Modern methods using polymerase chain reaction (PCR) techniques can detect very small quantities of viral nucleic acids but cannot determine if these nucleic acids are present in living viruses in the blood. So, detecting the time at which the virus first appears in the blood is not a simple task or one determined with any certainty.

after inoculation [Ryabchikova, 1994]. EBOV was detected in the blood of rhesus monkeys 24 hours after a subcutaneous injection with a dose of 10^5 PFU (this corresponds to at least 10^5 LD_{50}) [Fisher-Hoch, 1985]. ZEBOV was isolated from blood of a baboon 4 days after the subcutaneous inoculation of a dose of 20 LD_{50} [Luchko, 1995]. ZEBOV was found in the blood of rhesus monkeys 72 hours after aerosol exposure to a dose of 5 LD_{50} [Pyankov, 1995]. The time of appearance of the virus in the bloodstream appears to depend more on magnitude of the infectious dose and less on the inoculation route.

Primary Target Cells

Identifying the first target cell is difficult. The total number of cells in an organism is tremendous, and the number of initially infected cells is incomparably small. Based on our studies, we have calculated that the concentration of virus must be greater than 10^3 LD_{50}/mL in a 10% suspension of infected organ tissue to ensure reproducible detection by electron microscopy. One particle of EBOV or MARV has been calculated to be equivalent to one lethal dose for monkeys [Chermashentsev, 1993]. Studies of guinea pigs infected with mouse-adapted ZEBOV showed experimentally that one LD_{50} might be equal to one virus particle [Bray, 2001]. This means that one infectious dose is equal to one viral particle and that the one viral particle is able to infect one cell to start a deadly infection. This is an incredibly efficient process of viral entry and replication in host cells as each virus is able to initiate a productive infection. To circumvent these problems, we developed several experimental approaches to identify the primary target cells for ZEBOV and MARV infections.

Lymph Nodes

The first approach to identifying the primary target cells was based on the fact that most invading pathogens encounter lymph nodes, which act as filters for trapping microorganisms, as the first line of immune defense. We examined the possible entrapment of ZEBOV in lymph nodes of guinea pigs after intramuscular injection at a defined depth (0.5 cm). (The ZEBOV inoculum was from the green monkey liver suspension.) The injection site and the involved lymph nodes were examined at 1, 2, 4, 12, 24, and 48 hours after the inoculation using light and electron microscopy. We did not find any signs of viral reproduction at the injection site although the site was clearly identified by the presence of macrophages containing phagosomes with hepatic debris from the inoculum. These results suggest that ZEBOV is released rapidly from the inoculation site [Ryabchikova, 1999]. No signs of ZEBOV reproduction were found in the surrounding small lymph nodes and regional inguinal lymph node.

These findings are in contrast to published results examining the trapping of Salmonella flagellae by rat lymph nodes after footpad administration. The flagellae, which are similar in size to EBOV (about 1 μ in length), were detected in the regional lymph nodes within 3–4 minutes and were found to be entrapped there for 48 hours [Nossal, 1968]. Thus, since ZEBOV was not trapped in the lymph nodes, it must have infected the primary target cell very quickly, almost immediately after being injected into the tissue.

Injection Site Localization

In 1994, Skripchenko performed a set of experiments to test the hypothesis that the first infected cells might be localized at the injection site [Skripchenko, 1994]. If MARV is inoculated intraperitoneally, the cells in the highest concentrations in the peritoneum are likely to be the first infected; these are the mesothelial cells and macrophages. Macrophages are remarkably versatile and they take part in many physiological and pathological processes. They came into existence early during vertebrate evolution and have acquired numerous essential regulatory functions. Macrophages and neutrophils are sometimes referred to as "professional phagocytes" because both use phagocytosis to eliminate microorganisms from infected tissues. Other important roles of macrophages are in the immune system and anti-inflammatory response. The role of macrophage cells in filoviral disease pathogenesis will be considered in subsequent chapters of this book. Peritoneal macrophages normally are located on the surface of the peritoneal cavity. Their function is to regenerate the mesothelium layer bordering the cavity and to eliminate damaged cells, infections, and debris. The number of peritoneal macrophages increases in the case of any peritoneal inflammation (peritonitis).

Guinea pigs were infected intraperitoneally with 100 LD$_{50}$ of MARV (10% liver suspension) and peritoneal fluid was removed 1, 24, 48, and 72 hours after the infection. The PFU assay showed MARV replication in the cells of peritoneal exudate at 24, 48, and 72 hours post-inoculation, while the cells removed at 1 hour were not yet infected.

Electron microscopic studies of the same preparations showed evidence of MARV reproduction in the macrophage cells at 48 and 72 hours post-inoculation. Figure 4-1 shows viral replication in a macrophage cell of the peritoneal fluid taken from infected guinea pigs. Two viral inclusion areas can be seen with the characteristic circular cross-section shapes of MARV. In addition, several viral particles were seen outside of the plasma membrane of the macrophage. Neutrophils, monocytes, and lymphoid cells in the samples showed no visible morphological evidence of viral infection. Examination of the mesothelium cells also showed no signs

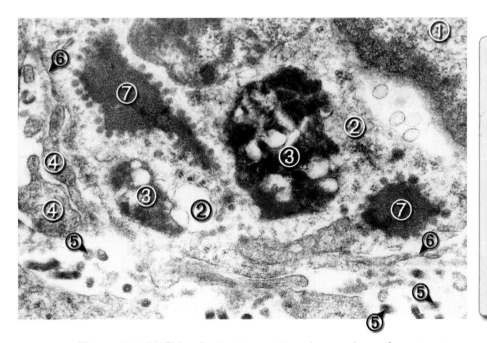

Legend

Figure 4-1

1. Nucleus
2. Cytoplasm
3. Phagosome
4. Macrophage protrusion
5. Viral particle
6. Plasma membrane
7. Viral inclusion body

See Note on page xiii.

Figure 4-1. MARV replication in a peritoneal macrophage of a guinea pig as seen in an ultrathin section of the cells of peritoneal exudate obtained at 72 h post-inoculation (magnification 31,000). Peritoneal macrophages are on the surface of the peritoneal cavity. These macrophages eliminate damaged cells and are located on the mesotheluim layer. The filoviruses are able to replicate in these cells. Even the virion budding is seen around the viral inclusions.

of viral infection. Based on these results, only the macrophage cells in the peritoneal fluid appeared infected.

Macrophage Cells and Susceptibility

Since the macrophages are definitely a target for MARV, differences in cultured macrophage cells' ability to support viral replication could reflect differences in the virus' ability to infect an intact host. Skripchenko studied MARV reproduction *in vitro* in peritoneal macrophage cells [Skripchenko, 1991]. Macrophages were isolated from the peritoneal cavity of rabbits, guinea pigs, green monkeys, rhesus monkeys, and baboons. Macrophage cells were also obtained from ascites fluid from humans with cardiovascular diseases. Ascites fluid (an abnormal accumulation of serous fluid in the abdominal cavity) was removed from patients in the course of standard treatment at the Novosibirsk region hospital. The macrophage cells were collected by centrifugation and were used for these experiments.

The cultured macrophage cells were infected with 0.1 PFU/cell of MARV after 2 days of propagation. These infected macrophages were cultured at 37 °C for 9 days. The supernatants were tested for MARV at 1 hour post-inoculation and then daily from 1 to 9 days post-inoculation by PFU assay and compared. If no plaques were detected after 9 days, this meant there were no viruses in the sample. From the results presented in Tables 4-2 and 4-3, MARV reproduction in peritoneal macrophages differs between animal species.

The growth of MARV in macrophages was divided into three groups:

1. High: man, guinea pigs, and green monkeys.
2. Intermediate (with marked differences between individuals): rhesus monkeys and baboons.*
3. Negative (MARV growth not detected): rabbits.

These results are consistent with other research examining the susceptibility of species to MARV infection. In 1996, Peters showed that guinea pigs, green monkeys, and rhesus monkeys are highly susceptible to MARV [Peters, 1996]. Our preliminary studies showed that baboons are less susceptible to the virus and in

---

*Three different baboons were used to provide peritoneal macrophages. Each of these macrophage cells was infected and the propagation of filoviruses in these cells was measured. Two cultures of these infected macrophage cells had virus titers similar to humans, but the cells from one of the baboons never showed infection over the 9 days.

Table 4-2. MARV titers (PFU) in peritoneal macrophage cultured medium from various animals.

	Time After Inoculation									
	1 hour	1 day	2 days	3 days	4 days	5 days	6 days	7 days	8 days	9 days
Animals Studied	MARV Titers (PFU) in Peritoneal Macrophage*									
Humans[†]	0[‡]	2.34	2.77	3.04	NS[§]	3.54	NS	5.14	5.22	5.67
Guinea pigs	0	NS	3.56	4.51	4.80	4.71	5.58	NS	NS	NS
Green monkeys	0	NS	4.25	5.19	5.34	5.51	4.59	4.54	4.48	NS
Rhesus monkeys	0	0	0	0	0	0.68	2.80	2.68	3.3	2.18
Rabbits	0	0	0	0	0	0	0	0	0	0

* PFU in $\log_{10}$
[†] Average of four human donors
[‡] Plaques were not detected
[§] NS – No sample

Table 4-3. MARV titers (PFU) in peritoneal macrophage cultured medium from baboons.

	Time After Inoculation									
	1 hour	1 day	2 days	3 days	4 days	5 days	6 days	7 days	8 days	9 days
Animals Studied	MARV Titers (PFU) in Peritoneal Macrophage*									
Baboon #1	0[†]	0	0	0	0	0	0	0	0	0
Baboon #2	0	NS[‡]	2.44	2.72	3.23	3.46	3.66	NS	NS	4.26
Baboon #3	0	2.18	2.97	4.36	4.9	4.9	NS	4.98	5.39	5.66

* PFU in $\log_{10}$
[†] Plaques were not detected
[‡] NS – No sample

fact, they occasionally show asymptomatic courses of disease. Rabbits are resistant to MARV since even infection with 10^7 LD_{50} did not produce clinical disease; however, the rabbits did produce virus-specific antibodies. These results also indicated that the animals' susceptibility to infections is related to the ability of the macrophage to support filoviral replication. Thus, the macrophages can be used as indicators of a species' susceptibility to MARV.

We used time course studies of filovirus-infected guinea pigs and green monkeys to gain more evidence for the involvement of macrophage cells in the first steps of filoviral infections. We again used intraperitoneal inoculation with filoviruses but looked at the liver, one of the known target organs for MARV. In one set of experiments, we inoculated guinea pigs and green monkeys intraperitoneally with MARV at a dose of 100 LD_{50}. The first infected cells were resident hepatic macrophages (Kuppfer cells) that were found on day 3 after IP inoculation. In green monkeys infected with ZEBOV at the same dose, macrophages were also the first infected cells and they were found in the lumen of hepatic blood vessels 2 days after inoculation [Ryabchikova, 1994; Ryabchikova, 1998]. A Kuppfer cell infected with ZEBOV is shown in Figure 4-2. It confirms that ZEBOV can replicate in macrophage cells. The typical cross-section pattern of ZEBOV nucleocapsids in viral inclusions near the nucleus and phago-somes are visible. Individual nucleocapsids are also visible, but these could be confused with the ER membrane at the low magnification. The Kuppfer cells normally eliminate bacteria, viruses, and other infectious agents, as well as many waste products. However, the filovirus is able to replicate in these cells and subsequently infect other cells, including hepatocytes. Other researchers have confirmed that Ebola replicates in macrophages; this has been noted in subsequent publications [Davis, 1997; Connolly, 1999; Geisbert, 1998].

Guinea pigs did not die after inoculation with fresh isolates of ZEBOV obtained from humans or monkeys (non-adapted ZEBOV). However, the virus caused acute disease with fever and focal hepatic inflammation. Samples of visceral organs from guinea pigs infected with ZEBOV were taken daily; on day 7, we noted the first signs of viral reproduction in hepatic monocyte-

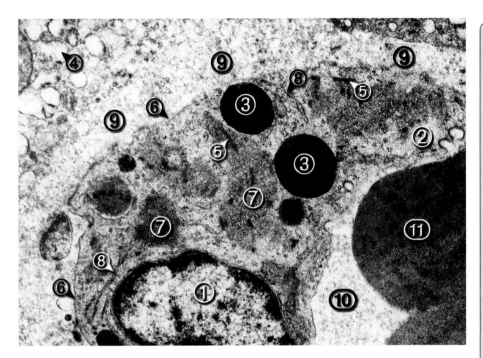

Legend

Figure 4-2
1. Nucleus
2. Cytoplasm
3. Phagosome
4. Hepatocyte
5. Viral nucleocapsid
6. Kuppfer cell membrane
7. Viral inclusion
8. Endoplasmic reticulum (ER)
9. Disse's space
10. Sinusoid lumen
11. Erythrocyte

See Note on page xiii.

Figure 4-2. An ultrathin section of a Kuppfer (macrophage) cell in a liver of green monkey infected by ZEBOV, day 3 post-inoculation (magnification 20,000). The electron microscope picture confirms that ZEBOV replicates in the Kuppfer cells. The viral inclusions are clearly visible.

macrophage cells. During the 21 days of infection, none of the other cellular targets were involved in ZEBOV reproduction in guinea pigs [Ryabchikova, 1996]. The results of all these experiments again indicate that the macrophage is the primary target for MARV and ZEBOV in monkeys and guinea pigs.

In filoviral pathogenesis, the first action of the filovirus is to replicate in the macrophages and produce progeny virus. The primary infected macrophages release the progeny virus into the bloodstream or lymph flow, which subsequently transports the virions throughout the organism. Migration of the infected macrophages into the parenchyma and interstitial tissue is another way of virus dissemination. We detected the passage of infected macrophages through blood vessel walls in sections of lymph nodes of ZEBOV-infected monkeys. Macrophages that enter the parenchyma or interstitial tissue can then release viral particles into the surrounding space, thereby infecting the adjacent cells. Obviously, infected macrophages can leave the bloodstream or lymphatic flow to reach any compartment of the organism. In fact, we detected infected macrophages in all the visceral organs that we studied in monkeys and guinea pigs, including the pancreas, esophagus, intestines, salivary glands, and heart. Interestingly, the heart parenchyma cells were not observed to support filoviral reproduction. Our data on the localization of filovirus-infected macrophages in interstitial tissue of visceral organs are in good agreement with results and findings published elsewhere. The presence of infected macrophages in interstitial tissue has been demonstrated in green and cynomolgus monkeys at the terminal stages of Ebola and Marburg diseases [Geisbert, 1992; Jaax, 1996; Johnson, 1995; Murphy, 1971]. The localization of the infected macrophages in all the visceral organs in MARV- and EBOV-infected animals is the reason why the filoviruses are regarded as pantropic viruses (i.e., viruses that have an affinity for affecting many kinds of tissue). The role of macrophages in providing resistance or susceptibility to filoviral infection is further investigated in Chapter 5.

Aerosol Infection

We also attempted to identify the primary target cells for filoviruses following aerosol exposure to MARV. If macrophage cells are the primary target cells, then infected macrophages should be present in the lung after aerosol exposure to the virus. Guinea pigs were exposed to aerosolized MARV at a dose of 2–5 LD_{50} and pulmonary lavages were obtained at 16, 24, 32, 40, 48, and 56 hours post-inoculation. Using PFU assays, evidence of viral reproduction was found in the lavages at 40 hours post-inoculation. Electron microscopic studies of the lavaged cells revealed MARV inclusions and nucleocapsids in the macrophage cells [Ryabchikova, 1996a]. Evidence of MARV reproduction was also found in pulmonary lavages obtained at 32 hours post-inoculation from aerosol-challenged rhesus monkeys, using the PFU assay [Pyankov, 1995]. The results of aerosol experiments revealed that the primary targets for MARV are the macrophage cells.

Secondary Target Cells

Time course studies of the visceral organs revealed other cellular targets for MARV and ZEBOV. Hepatocytes were the second infected target cells found in ZEBOV- and MARV-infected monkeys on day 3–4 post-inoculation. These cells can be infected by the viral particles released from the primary infected Kuppfer cells. Large numbers of filoviral particles were produced by hepatocytes that occupy the space between the hepatocytes and sinusoids (Disse's spaces [DS]). This can be seen in Figure 4-3. The MARV-infected hepatocyte is shown in Figure 4-3A. The viral particles and viral inclusions are clearly visible. A ZEBOV-infected hepatocyte cell is shown in Figure 4-3B. The viral inclusions of ZEBOV nucleocapsids are also apparent.

During infection, the number of filovirus-infected hepatocytes and therefore the number of virions produced increases. The hepatocytes are good hosts because of their large capacity for protein synthesis. Filoviral infection alters the hepatic functions and, consequently, the level of toxic materials in the blood increases and causes further damage to the circulatory system. Circulatory shock and poor perfusion add to the damage done to the liver. Examination of the liver sections showed that the virions remain in the hepatic parenchyma, mostly in the area bordered by hepatocytes and the sinusoid wall. These virions are eventually released into the blood late in the course of the disease and only after the sinusoid walls have been completely destroyed. Thus, although the liver is a site of active filoviral reproduction, it is not prominent in the further dissemination of the virus; numerous progeny virions remain in the parenchyma and are not engaged in the spread of the infection.

ZEBOV reproduction was also found in green monkey adrenal cortical cells on days 4 to 5 post-inoculation. Both the viral inclusions and individual viral particles can be seen in Figure 4-4. The adrenal glands are small but play an important role by secreting vital hormones. The adrenal cortex is responsible for producing glucocorticoids, which, among other functions, have anti-inflammatory properties. The adrenal cortical cells are the other type of parenchymal cells (in addition to hepatocytes) that are able to support MARV and ZEBOV replication. The

Figure 4-3A

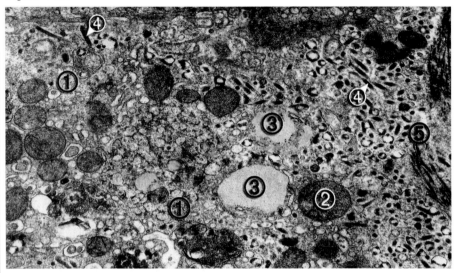

Legend

Figure 4-3

1. Cytoplasm
2. Mitochondria
3. Lipid droplet
4. Viral particle
5. Disse's space
6. Viral inclusion
   body
7. Nucleus

See Note on page xiii.

Figure 4-3B

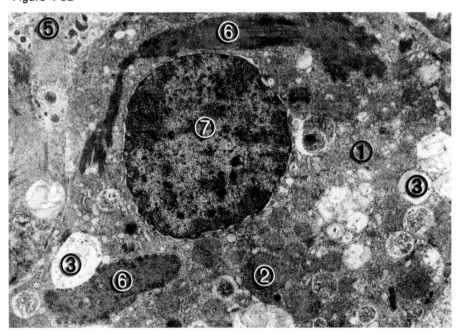

Figure 4-3. Ultrathin sections showing replication of filoviruses in hepatocytes of green monkeys. Hepatocytes have large capacities for protein synthesis, making them good hosts for filoviral replication. After infecting Kuppfer cells, filoviruses reproduce in large quantities, which alters normal liver functions and in turn causes increased concentrations of toxic material in the blood and eventual damage to the circulation system and other organs. **Figure 4-3A** shows MARV-infected hepatocytes of a green monkey (magnification 12,000). **Figure 4-3B** shows ZEBOV-infected hepatocytes of a green monkey (magnification 8,000).

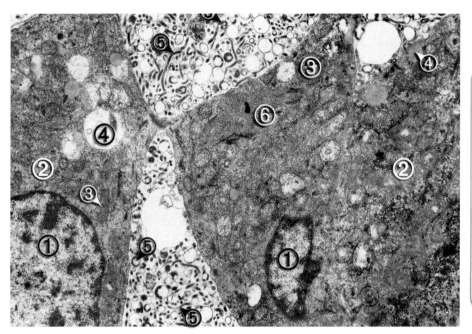

Legend

Figure 4-4
1. Nucleus
2. Cytoplasm
3. Mitochondria
4. Lipid droplet
5. Viral particle
6. Viral inclusion body

See Note on page xiii.

Figure 4-4. Ultrathin section of adrenal cortex showing replication of ZEBOV in green monkey adrenal cortical cells (magnification 7,000). Filoviral infection in the adrenal glands alters general hormone production in animals. (Photo by Dr. L. Kolesnikova)

morphological features of filoviral infections are similar in infected adrenal cortical cells and hepatocytes. In REBOV-infected cynomolgus monkeys, virus reproduction was found not only in the adrenal cortical cell, but also in the adrenal medulla cells [Geisbert, 1992].

The involvement of cells in filoviral infection depends, at least, on their ability to support viral replication and their accessibility to the virus. Virions produced by primary infected macrophages are delivered to all organs by blood and lymph. Since the filovirus is then in close proximity to endothelial cells, it is quite reasonable to expect that endothelial cells should be at least the secondary targets for the filoviruses. Endothelial cells make up capillaries and post-capillary veins and form borders between the blood or lymph and surrounding tissue. In support of the expectation that endothelial cells are secondary targets, experiments *in vitro* demonstrated that MARV and EBOV replicate in cultured human endothelial cells [Schnittler, 1993; Gupta, 2001]. Our animal experiments show that infected endothelial cells can be found only at the late stages of the disease, usually during the 2 days before death [Ryabchikova, 1994; Ryabchikova, 1999; Ryabchikova, 1999a]. In spite of the presence of viremia, we observed very few infected endothelial cells from days 5 to 6 post-inoculation in green monkeys infected with MARV and ZEBOV. Figures 4-5A and 4-5B show viral inclusions in the endothelial cells and therefore indicate that both ZEBOV and MARV can replicate in these cells. Although rare, infected endothelial cells were found in all the examined visceral organs in monkeys and guinea pigs before death. Other researchers have reported filovirus-infected endothelial cells, but even though animals were inoculated at high doses, infected cells

Figure 4-5A

Legend

Figure 4-5

1. Cytoplasm
2. Blood vessel lumen
3. Collagen fiber
4. Fibroblast
5. Viral inclusion body
6. Viral particle

See Note on page xiii.

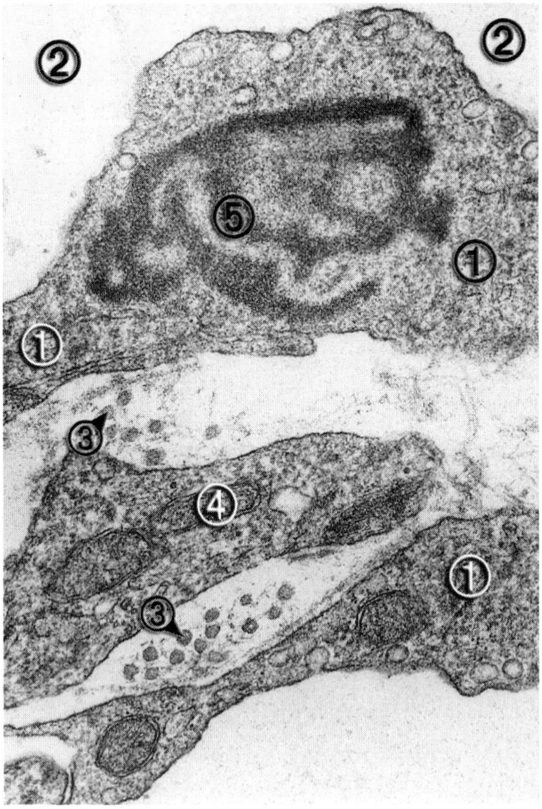

Figure 4-5. Ultrathin sections showing replication of filoviruses in green monkey endothelial cells. Very few infected endothelial cells are observed even late in the course of the infections. **Figure 4-5A** is from a MARV-infected green monkey (magnification 37,000). **Figure 4-5B** is from a ZEBOV-infected green monkey (magnification 26,000).

only appeared in small numbers from day 6 post-inoculation [Baskerville, 1985; Davis, 1997; Jaax, 1996; Johnson, 1995; Murphy, 1971]. Thus, in spite of the access of viruses to endothelial cells from the very first days of infection, endothelial cells are infected late in the disease and the number of infected cells is small. While their role in viral production appears less important, the altered function of endothelial cells cannot be ignored.

Fibroblasts are also expected to be target cells. These are located in the interstitial tissue of all the visceral organs, and they are adjacent to the infected macrophages. Fibroblasts have long thin protrusions that can pass the budding filoviruses far from the cell. This can be seen in the ZEBOV-infected fibroblast of a rhesus

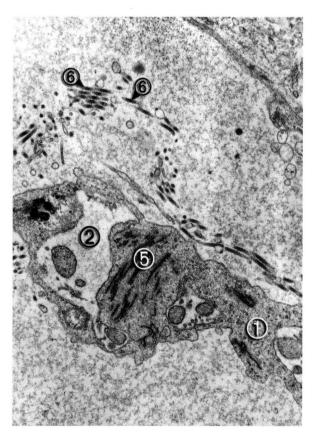

Figure 4-5B

monkey, shown in Figures 4-6A and B. Infected fibroblasts disseminate filoviruses within the tissues using these protrusions. Davis emphasized the significance of infected fibroblasts for local spreading of filoviruses. The infected fibroblasts and interstitial macrophages lay in the interstitial tissue and their viral progeny did not enter the bloodstream [Davis, 1997].

Legend

Figure 4-6

1. Lymphocyte
2. Macrophage
3. Budding virion
4. Nucleocapsid
5. Fibroblast plasma membrane
6. Viral inclusion
7. Interstitial tissue
8. Viral particle
9. Endoplasmic reticulum (ER)
10. Collagen
11. Fibroblast protrusion

See Note on page xiii.

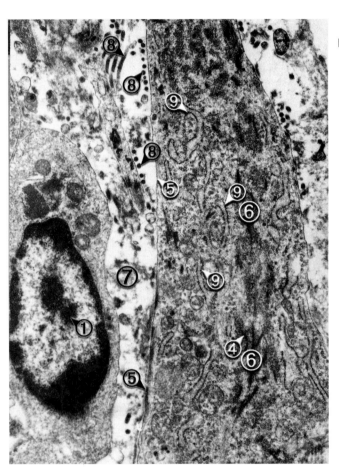

Figure 4-6A

Figure 4-6. Ultrathin sections showing replication of ZEBOV in fibroblasts of rhesus monkey. Fibroblasts are the main elements of connective tissues. They produce collagen and have large capacities for protein synthesis, which the virus may use for replication. Fibroblasts can also help to disseminate filoviruses using their protrusions to reach beyond the immediate cell area. **Figure 4-6A** shows the central part of fibroblast body and neighboring lymphocyte (magnification 10,000). **Figure 4-6B** shows the protrusion of an infected fibroblast and budding virions (magnification 15,000).

Other Target Cells

In our studies, all target cells for filoviral infections are identifiable from day 5 post-inoculation and include the following: macrophages, hepatocytes, adrenal cortical cells, endothelial cells, and fibroblasts. As we observed in our monkey studies, occasionally other cells also can be involved in filoviral reproduction. These other cells were found very rarely and in single animals, but they deserve attention. These other cells are alveolar cells and epithelial cells of bronchi in ZEBOV-infected monkeys, and the cells of the endocardial layer. Alveolar epithelial cells and the ciliated cells of the bronchial lining were infected in some of the green

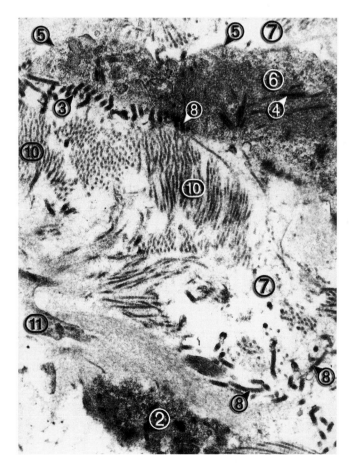

Figure 4-6B

monkeys and are shown in Figure 4-7. Both viral particles and viral inclusions can be seen. Another researcher has reported REBOV reproduction in rare alveolar cells, in epithelial cells of renal proximal tubules, and in cells of the adrenal medulla [Geisbert, 1992]. The mechanisms that provide viral reproduction in all

Figure 4-7A

Legend

Figure 4-7

1. Nucleus
2. Cytoplasm
3. Basal membrane
4. Alveolar cell plasma membrane
5. Viral particle
6. Viral inclusion body
7. Collagen
8. Blood vessel
9. Cilia
10. Alveolar space
11. Nucleocapsid

See Note on page xiii.

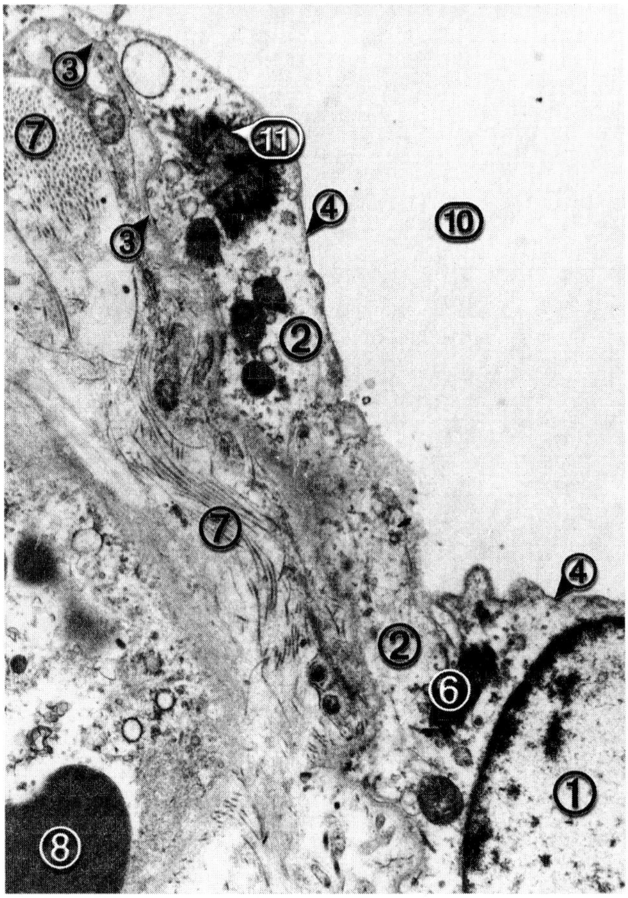

Figure 4-7. ZEBOV replication occurs rarely in the airway cells of green monkeys. The airway epithelium is a cellular layer responsible for air cleaning, humidifying, and gas exchange. Usually filoviruses do not reproduce in the lung epithelium, and only a few infected monkeys showed a rare replication of ZEBOV and MARV in the bronchial and alveoli cells. **Figure 4-7A** shows a ZEBOV-infected alveolar epithelial cell (type I) (magnification 11,000). **Figure 4-7B** shows ZEBOV-infected ciliated cells of bronchial lining (magnification 8,000). (Photos by Dr. L. Kolesnikova)

the various types of cells are still unknown. The ability of EBOV to infect the cells of respiratory pathways should be examined because if the respiratory pathways can be infected, it is possible that EBOV can be spread as a respiratory disease. This is incomparably more dangerous than the existing model of disease spread via contact with body fluids.

Our examination of the visceral organs following the aerosol MARV inoculation of guinea pigs revealed the same sequence and pattern of cell involvement in viral reproduction as in green monkeys. We identified macrophages as the primary targets. Hepatocytes, fibroblasts, and endothelial cells were involved in viral reproduction but at later stages of the infection.

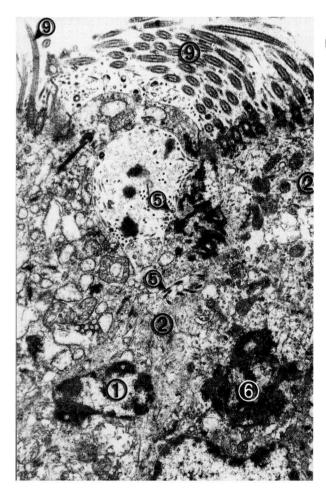

Figure 4-7B

There is a set of cellular targets that we never found to be infected in experimental animals, and these should be mentioned. Unlike earlier reports, which indicated filoviruses replicated in lymphocytes [Baskerville, 1985], in all the animals we studied, we found no evidence of MARV and ZEBOV reproduction in lymphocytes and neutrophils. This is in agreement with other researchers who also noted that lymphocytes were not infected by filoviruses, even using *in situ* hybridization and immunochemistry [Geisbert, 1992; Jaax, 1996; Davis, 1997; Geisbert, 1998]. This finding is very helpful in clarifying the pathogenic mechanisms. It indicates that in filoviral infections, disturbances in the immune system organs and functions are not related to viral reproduction in lymphocytes and neutrophils. Recent studies on interactions of pseudotyped murine leukemia virus containing the glycoprotein from ZEBOV confirmed the inability of ZEBOV to infect lymphatic cells [Wool-Lewis, 1998]. Filoviruses also do not reproduce in nerve cells, smooth and striated muscle cells, or in the epithelial layer of intestines and stomach. We did not find filoviral reproduction in pancreatic cells in monkeys and guinea pigs. This is a contradiction with observations that MARV had a "predilection for viral infection of pancreatic islet cells," as noted in a human who died after MARV infection [Geisbert, 1998]. This difference may be related to differences in surface receptors on pancreatic cells in animals and humans.

Conclusion

We were able to correlate the susceptibility of different animal species with the susceptibility of their macrophages to support filoviral growth. And we were able to identify the target cell for filoviral infections in the intact host as the macrophage. The time course studies revealed the following sequence of the cell involvement in viral reproduction in MARV- and ZEBOV-infected animals: macrophages, hepatocytes, adrenal cortical cells, endothelial cells, and fibroblasts. These same cells (macrophages, hepatocytes, adrenal cortical cells, endothelial cells, and fibroblasts) have been reported as target cells by other authors who examined the organs of ZEBOV- and MARV-infected monkeys before death [Baskerville, 1985; Davis, 1997; Jaax, 1996; Johnson,

1995; Murphy, 1971]. Identical target cells were found in cynomolgus monkeys infected with REBOV [Geisbert, 1992]. The Sudan strain of EBOV, SEBOV, has been poorly studied. Viral particles were identified in the monkey liver and spleen, but target cells were not described and identified [Ellis, 1978; Fisher-Hoch, 1992]. Our data are unique because no other investigators, to our knowledge, have conducted daily examinations of the visceral organs in filovirus-infected monkeys. One other study did use daily tissue samples to study the disease progression in ZEBOV-infected guinea pigs; however, this study used $10^{3.8}$ PFU ZEBOV/0.5 mL inoculated subcutaneously [Connolly, 1999] and would not be sensitive enough to notice the organism's defensive reactions as they come into play. Recently, a serial sacrifice study of ZEBOV adapted to BALB/c mice was also published [Gibb, 2001] and confirmed macrophages as the targets. The mice were inoculated with 100 PFU (3000 LD_{50}), much higher than the dose we used in our experiments (1–200 LD_{50}, Table 2-1).

The total number of filovirus-infected cells depends on the time after inoculation. We examined visceral organs of green and rhesus monkeys (which died on days 7 and 8 post-inoculation), in baboons (which died on days 9–10), and in cynomolgus monkeys (which died on days 10–14). Our studies demonstrated the same set of target cells as in the time course studies for ZEBOV in the four monkey species.

The total number of infected cells and viral particles in the sections from the examined organs was the greatest in cynomolgus monkeys. We were able to frequently observe infected endothelial cells and fibroblasts in the organs of cynomolgus monkeys but rarely observed infected endothelial cells in the other monkey species. Obviously, the longer disease course provides more opportunities for ZEBOV to infect larger numbers of cells. So paradoxically, at least at the beginning of the disease, the longer the animal lives, the larger the number of virus progeny that accumulate in the organs; however, this accumulation does not determine lethality. Rhesus and green monkeys had significantly fewer infected cells, but they died a week earlier than cynomolgus monkeys.

For those not familiar with the use of electron microscopy in viral studies, it is worth repeating that the observations of viral particles and lesions require very careful sample selection and preparation. We examined many light microscope samples looking for viral structures and damage from viral infections, and we selected our electron microscopy samples from these areas. When we say that a feature was rarely found, it means that we looked at hundreds of light microscopy samples and hundreds of electron microscope photos and only saw the feature a few times. As an analogy, using electron microscopy would be similar to looking for a specific house on a large map of a large city, but viewing the map through a filter the size of a pinhead.

Filoviral reproduction in animal cells is the major event in the pathogenesis of the disease and determines the fatality. We identified a set of filovirus-infected cells and the sequence of their involvement during the course of infections in experimentally inoculated animals. Based on our time course studies, we developed a model for the replication and dissemination of the filoviruses in monkeys and guinea pigs during infection. This is shown in the schematic in Figure 4-8. The first step is the infection of macrophages, and then the filovirus-infected macrophages are carried through the blood and lymph systems to the secondary target cells, where filoviral reproduction again occurs. This is the point of secondary infection; subsequently, the filovirus-infected macrophages, but not the other virus-infected cells, are carried in the blood and lymph to all organs. Having established that macrophages are infected first and are the predominant cells spreading the infection in the body, our next step in the study of filoviral pathogenesis is to examine the nature of pathological changes in the visceral organs and how these changes are related to filoviral replication.

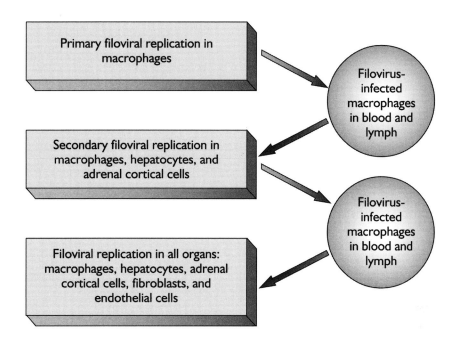

Figure 4-8. Sequential steps of filoviral dissemination during infections in guinea pigs and monkeys. This schematic emphasizes the spread of filoviruses from the sites of virus replication via blood and lymph from infected macrophages. While other types of cells may support filoviral replication, the dissemination is done almost exclusively by the infected macrophages.

chapter 5

Microscopic Pathology over the Course of Filoviral Infection

The first step in understanding the course of any infectious disease is identifying the pathogen and then determining the course of the disease produced by the pathogen in an appropriate animal model. By understanding how the disease develops, and how the pathogen affects the various critical organs in an animal or human, various strategies can be used to prevent or treat the disease. In viral diseases, a principal component is understanding viral reproduction or replication. Particularly important is the determination of which tissues support replication and what happens to those tissues as a result of viral growth. Additionally, viruses can cause changes in cells even though viral reproduction does not occur in those cells. These changes often occur through disturbances in normal biochemical processes or alterations in the immune system functions. Thus, pathological changes in various tissues and organs can develop both directly from viral infections of and replications in the cells and indirectly from changes in other cells and their functions. Those organs in which these changes occur are the target organs. In this chapter, we examine filoviral replication in various types of cells in the visceral organs of infected animals. In Chapter 7, "Time Course of the Pathological Changes in Filovirus-Infected Animals," we will examine the organ pathology of each of these target organs.

We examined the visceral organs of monkeys infected with 10^5 LD_{50} of MARV and ZEBOV. At the terminal stages, necrosis was pronounced in the target organs; sometimes necrosis was so advanced that the tissue architecture was completely lost. As we will discuss in Chapter 7, some of the necrosis is undoubtedly due to poor perfusion and changes in permeability of the blood vessels and thrombosis. Many viral particles were seen in the cells of the liver and lymphatic organs. The pattern of pathological changes was the same in different monkey species and for both MARV and ZEBOV infections. The descriptions are similar to observations from human autopsy studies [Zaki, 1997]. This similarity in pathological changes in the organs between monkeys and humans is a strong argument for using monkey models in investigations of filoviral pathogenesis.

Previous publications dealing with the morphological changes in visceral organs of filovirus-infected animals described the pathology late in the disease in animals inoculated with large infectious doses (10^5 LD_{50}) [Baskerville, 1978; Baskerville, 1985; Fisher-Hoch, 1992; Geisbert, 1992; Jaax, 1996; Johnson, 1995; Siegert, 1972]. These descriptions primarily came from post-mortem examinations. In our work, we have been fortunate to be able to examine animal tissues and cells at varying stages of the disease, not just at the terminal stage.

Experimental Design

In order to understand how the disease develops, we followed the time course of filoviral replication and pathological changes in infected animals. We chose the guinea pig and green monkey as the species to study because of their high susceptibility to ZEBOV and MARV (Table 4-2). We performed daily studies of the visceral organs, which had been identified as targets in the earlier post-mortem studies cited above. The goal was to establish those alterations in viral reproduction and organ morphology that were common to MARV and ZEBOV infections; further, once these alterations were established, we wanted to study the changes that develop during the progression of the infection. We also wanted to determine if the changes were uniform for all routes of infection or whether they would vary with the inoculation route. Complete descriptions of all the methods are given in Chapter 2, "Materials and Methods," but the pertinent experiments are summarized in Table 5-1.

Table 5-1. Summary of experimental design.

Series 1— Species Difference	Series 2— IP vs. Inhalation	Series 3— ZEBOV vs. MARV	Series 4— Course of Infection
Guinea pigs and green monkeys were inoculated with 100 LD$_{50}$ of MARV intraperitoneally (IP) to analyze for species-specific differences	Guinea pigs were inoculated with 2–5 LD$_{50}$ of MARV by the aerosol inhalation route to compare the infection pattern with that of the IP mode (these data were compared with those of Series 1)	Green monkeys were inoculated with 100 LD$_{50}$ of ZEBOV by the subcutaneous (SC) mode and compared with the infection course for MARV (Series 1)	Green monkeys were inoculated with 100 LD$_{50}$ of ZEBOV by either the IP, SC, or intratracheal modes, or via gastric tube into the stomach to examine the relation between the course of the infection and inoculation route

Post-inoculation samples were obtained daily for microscopic studies in Series 1, 2, and 3; samples for Series 4 were obtained only after the animals became moribund. Liver, spleen, lymph nodes (and lymphatic tissue from the intestines and lungs), kidneys, adrenals, lungs, heart, small and large intestines, pancreas, and salivary glands were all examined by light and electron microscopy.

The results showed that the progression of disease produced by filoviruses, as well as the observed organ pathology, were very similar in the green monkeys and guinea pigs from Series 1 and 2. However, in guinea pigs challenged by the aerosol route (Series 2), changes were observed 2 to 3 days later than when the guinea pigs were inoculated by the IP mode. This delay was consistently observed in all the examined organs, and to avoid redundancy, this fact is not repeated in each of the separate descriptions of organ damage. The patterns of pathological changes were the same regardless of the route of inoculation for green monkeys infected with the same doses of ZEBOV (Series 4). This pattern was the same as that observed for both the terminal stages of ZEBOV and MARV infections in green monkeys (Series 3). The exception was green monkeys infected with ZEBOV by placing the virus into the stomach. These monkeys did not develop any signs of ZEBOV infection and remained healthy.

Filoviral Reproduction

We first focus on the features of filoviral infection common to the two different animal species and then on the species-specific differences. As we described in Chapter 4 "Filoviral Infections," the target cells for ZEBOV and MARV are macrophages, hepatocytes, adrenal cortical cells, fibroblasts, and endothelial cells. This section is designed to provide an overview of filoviral reproduction in each target organ in green monkeys and guinea pigs during the course of MARV and ZEBOV infections.

Blood System

The circulatory system in infected hosts serves as the main mechanism to disseminate the filoviruses. Chapter 6, "Blood Disorders in Filoviral Infections," contains a detailed description of the role of the circulatory system and will cover the various pathological changes in the circulatory system, its role in disseminating filoviruses, and the effects of the virus throughout the infected animal's circulatory system. The main source of replication (i.e., the production) of the filoviruses in blood is the macrophages, first and foremost the hepatic macrophages, and then bone marrow macrophages and lymphatic tissue macrophages. Viral particles appear in the blood from infected cells located in all blood-washed organs and tissues, including all cells having contact with blood or lymph flow (resident macrophages in spleen, lymph nodes, and follicles). Viral reproduction also takes place in circulating macrophages. Infected macrophages usually contain viral inclusions and the rare individual nucleocapsid. Figure 4-1 shows MARV replication in the peritoneal macrophage of a guinea pig. Figure 5-1 shows a ZEBOV-infected macrophage from a lymph node. Early in the infection, macrophages appear to maintain their normal cytological structure and contain phagosomes, lysosomes, and residual bodies in their cytoplasm. And then later in the infection, macrophages no longer have definitive structures in them and are destroyed. This is discussed further in Chapter 7, "Time Course of the Pathological Changes in Filovirus-Infected Animals."

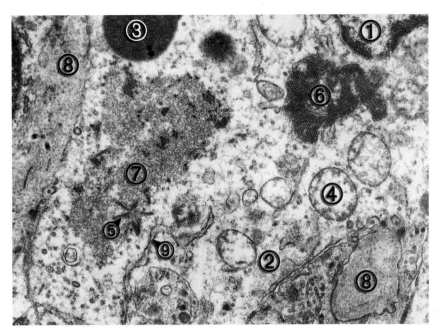

Legend

Figure 5-1
1. Nucleus
2. Cytoplasm
3. Phagosome
4. Mitochondria
5. Viral nucleocapsid
6. Interferon inclusion
7. Viral inclusion body
8. Intercellular space
9. Endoplasmic reticulum (ER)

See Note on page xiii.

Figure 5-1. An ultrathin section of macrophage infected with ZEBOV in a green monkey's lymphatic node (magnification 12,000). The macrophages in the lymphatic tissue are washed by lymph, which transports viral progeny to other sensitive cells and into the blood. The macrophage shown here is active in phagocytosis, as evidenced by the presence of a phagosome, and also in regulatory functions, as evidenced by the interferon crystalloid inclusion.

Despite the proximity of endothelial cells to filoviruses in blood vessels, they are not readily infected; evidence of MARV and ZEBOV infection was found in endothelial cells of the capillaries and venules only at the terminal stages of disease. Even then, the number of infected endothelial cells was small, and sometimes, no infected endothelial cells were observed, even in the presence of a great number of infected macrophages and hepatocytes in the liver. This is consistent with other researchers [Connolly, 1999] and is discussed in more detail in Chapter 6, "Blood Disorders in Filoviral Infections."

Liver

The liver is the main target organ for filoviruses, and filoviral reproduction produces marked damage to the hepatic structure and functions. We examined Kuppfer cells (resident macrophages in the liver), hepatocytes, fibroblasts, endothelial cells, leukocytes, and Ito cells (fat-containing cells located in Disse's space). In time course studies of guinea pigs and monkeys, the first filovirus-infected cells to be detected were the Kuppfer cells and circulating macrophages; these were found at days 2 to 3 after IP inoculation. This was described in Chapter 4. Evidence for filoviral infection in the hepatocytes was detected from day 4 post-inoculation, and each subsequent day the number of infected cells increased.

Infected hepatocytes were first found in the periportal zones, areas in which the blood first enters the liver. After this area, the infection spread throughout the lobules. Infected hepatocytes initially formed small foci of infection, whose size increased over time to include surrounding cells. In the terminal stages of disease, extensive areas of the hepatic parenchyma contained numerous cells with filovirus-specific structures. Figures 4-3A and 4-3B show MARV and ZEBOV replication in hepatocytes of green monkeys. Figure 5-2 shows virion budding from hepatocytes in a MARV-infected guinea pig. With large infectious doses, all the hepatocytes were infected within 4 to 5 days.

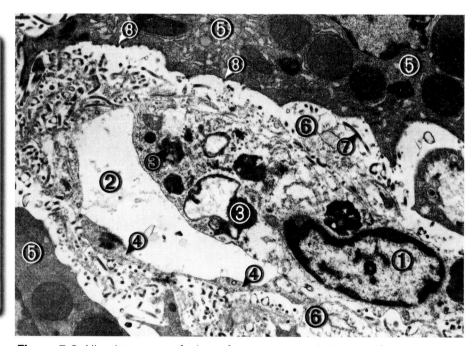

Legend

Figure 5-2

1. Nucleus of Kuppfer cell
2. Lumen of sinusoid
3. Phagosome
4. Endothelial cell
5. Hepatocyte
6. Disse's space
7. Viral particle
8. Budding virion on hepatocyte surface

See Note on page xiii.

Figure 5-2. Ultrathin section of a liver of guinea pig sampled 7 days after inoculation with MARV (magnification 11,000). The Kuppfer cells are the first infected cells; the viral particles are able to replicate in these resident hepatic macrophages. The new viral particles produced in the Kuppfer cells infect the adjacent hepatocytes and are transported by the blood to other cells and organs.

The viral inclusion bodies were usually found in the basal cytoplasm of the hepatocytes. MARV-infected hepatocytes contained small viral inclusions of irregular shape, while ZEBOV produced prominent inclusions, visible in a light microscope (see Figure 5-3), containing parallel arrays of packed nucleocapsids. These features can be seen in Figure 4-3B from a green monkey and in

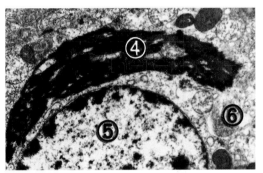

Figure 5-3B

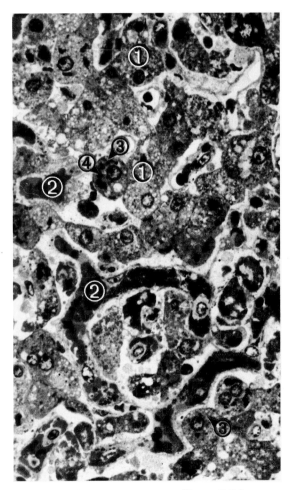

Figure 5-3A

Figure 5-3. Light and electron microscope views of ZEBOV-infected liver in a baboon. Sinusoids clogged by blood cells and some infected hepatocytes are seen. The cells were selected under the light microscope and then ultrathin sections were prepared for electron microscopy. **Figure 5-3A** (light microscope view) shows damage to the blood vessels where the sinusoids are clogged with blood cells. There is an absence of inflammation and dense inclusions are visible in the cytoplasm of some hepatocytes. **Figure 5-3B** (electron microscope view) represents a small area from Figure 5-3A and shows dense viral inclusions (magnification 6,000).

Legend

Figure 5-3

1. Hepatocyte
2. Sinusoid clogged with blood cells
3. Infected hepatocyte
4. Viral inclusion body
5. Nucleus
6. Cytoplasm

See Note on page xiii.

Figures 5-3 and 5-4A from a ZEBOV-infected baboon. Figure 5-4B shows hepatocytes from a MARV-infected guinea pig. The details of these infected hepatocytes and their effect on liver pathology are discussed further in Chapter 7, "Time Course of the Pathological Changes in Filovirus-Infected Animals."

The filoviruses bud on the basal and lateral plasma membranes of hepatocytes and never form on the apical plasma membrane, which borders the bile canaliculi. This budding pattern reflects the differences in the properties of the basal-lateral and apical plasma membranes of the hepatic cells. The same properties have been found in polarized epithelial Madin-Darby canine kidney (MDCK)

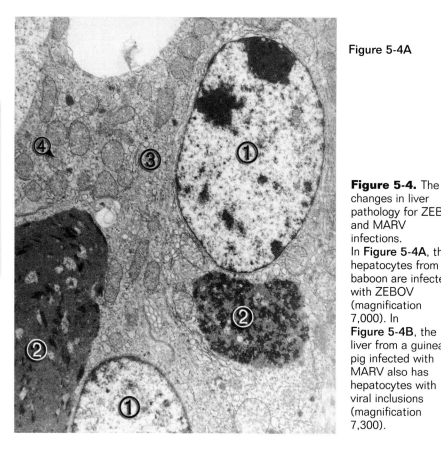

Figure 5-4A

Legend

Figure 5-4

1. Nucleus
2. Viral inclusion body
3. Cytoplasm
4. Mitochondria

See Note on page xiii.

Figure 5-4. The changes in liver pathology for ZEBOV and MARV infections. In **Figure 5-4A**, the hepatocytes from a baboon are infected with ZEBOV (magnification 7,000). In **Figure 5-4B**, the liver from a guinea pig infected with MARV also has hepatocytes with viral inclusions (magnification 7,300).

cells, where MARV particles are produced only on the basal-lateral surface [Sanger, 2001]. Infected hepatocytes produce large numbers of filoviral particles occupying the spaces between the neighboring cells, hepatocytes, and sinusoids (Disse's spaces); however, these viral particles remain inside the liver tissue and do not contribute to the viremia. As we discussed in Chapter 4, the formation of many large net-like spheres in the liver is typical for ZEBOV-infected animals. These net-like spheres can be seen in Figure 3-19. These net-like spheres are occasionally the only diagnostic feature that can be seen in the liver sections when only a few cells are infected with ZEBOV.

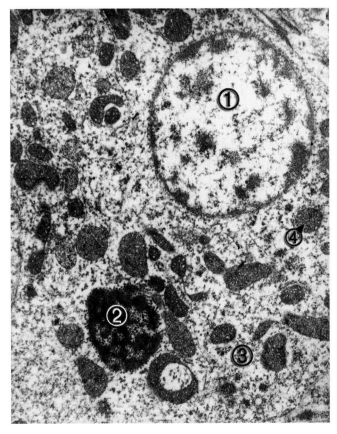

Figure 5-4B

Infected endothelial cells and fibroblasts are rarely detected in liver sections and then only in the last days of Marburg and Ebola viral disease. Figure 5-5 shows the typical viral inclusions and viral particles denoting an infected cell. The photograph is of an endothelial cell from the liver of a MARV-infected guinea pig. We did not find signs of MARV and ZEBOV reproduction in Ito cells in any of the infected animals.

We used both colony-reared and wild-caught monkeys in our studies of ZEBOV and MARV infections. The monkeys were clinically healthy (i.e., they did not show fever or other apparent signs of any disease). However, after the experiments, nonspecific pathologies (such as cirrhosis or severe dystrophy) from previous exposures to diseases or other agents were found during microscopic examination. The hepatocytes in infected and control

Legend

Figure 5-5

1. Nucleus of endothelial cell

2. Viral inclusion body

3. Lumen of sinusoid

4. Hepatocyte

5. Disse's space

6. Viral particle

See Note on page xiii.

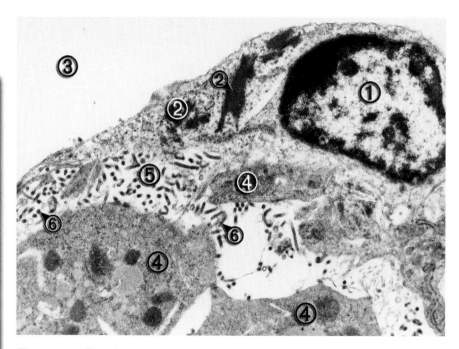

Figure 5-5. The ultrathin section of the liver of an infected guinea pig with the replication of MARV in the endothelial cell (magnification 11,300). The endothelial cells bordering the liver sinusoids transport substances arriving in the blood to the hepatocytes for detoxification. Filoviruses are able to infect the cells only at the late stages of infection. The total number of infected cells observed is usually very small, but even so, the involvement of the endothelial cells contributes to damaging hepatic functions.

(uninfected) monkeys showed various dystrophic changes (e.g., swelling of the mitochondria, vacuolization of the endoplasmic reticulum, lipid droplets, residual bodies, etc.). All the possible variations in pathological changes involving the cellular organelles in the liver were found in monkeys. Some of these changes were evident even in samples from control animals, and in those samples taken during the first 2 days post-inoculation (i.e., before the first signs of filoviral infections). Analysis of the samples showing nonspecific pathological changes revealed that altered hepatocytes were unable to produce complete MARV and ZEBOV virions. We rarely saw infected hepatocytes in these samples, but when we did, the viral inclusion bodies were not the typical filoviral shape. Figure 5-6 is an electron micrograph of an ultrathin section sample taken from tissues with altered hepatocytes and shows very dense viral and irregular-shaped ZEBOV inclusions, indicative of defective viral particles (i.e., virions without nucleocapsids). For comparison, see Figures 4-2 and 4-3b, both of which show examples of normal viral inclusions.* Although the hepatic parenchyma in these animals was not involved in filoviral reproduction, morphological signs of infection were consistently found only in hepatic macrophages. Sometimes it was impossible to find infected hepatocytes in livers that had nonspecific changes; only infected macrophages and fibroblasts were observed. However, the monkeys in whose livers the filovirus did not reproduce died from filoviral infection, as did monkeys with healthy livers. Thus, liver damage is not crucial to filoviral pathogenesis. This is consistent with clinical observations in human filoviral disease; hepatic impairment was not critical in the pathogenesis of filovirus-infected humans [Martini, 1971; Rippey, 1976; Simpson, 1980].

Special Note: Not all filoviral infections in hepatocytes are productive. Typically we found only the viral inclusions with no mature virion formation. The inclusion material may be very electron dense, showing no subtle details. If these hepatocytes produce viral particles, the particles are defective. We suggest that these cells illustrate unproductive variants of filoviral reproduction, presumably resulting from the failure of these hepatocytes to provide essential materials for viral synthesis. MARV and EBOV do not produce productive infections in hepatocytes that show prominent pathological changes of their structure, especially those structures that ordinarily support viral reproduction.

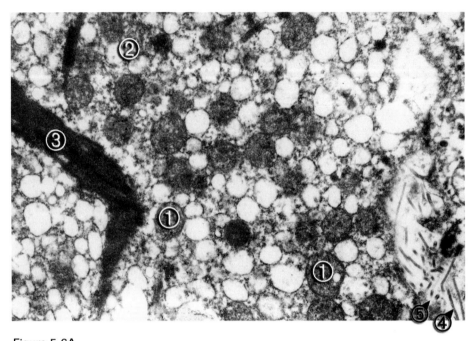

Figure 5-6A

Legend

Figure 5-6

1. Mitochondria

2. Cytoplasm

3. Viral inclusion
   body

4. Viral particle

5. Area of budding

See Note on page xiii.

Figure 5-6. Ultrathin sections highlighting differences from the normal replication of ZEBOV in the hepatocyte of a rhesus monkey. Ideally, pathogen-free animals would be used for filoviral (and indeed all viral) studies. However, there are no pathogen-free organisms in nature and despite using clinically healthy animals, some of the animal livers, including those from the control animals, had obvious pathologies. This is not uncommon nor should it affect our understanding of disease development in nature. All evolutionary events develop on the background of many parasite-host interactions. If we want to understand natural events and infections, we should examine natural systems, including animals having pathological changes. In this particular case, the ultrathin sections show that the altered hepatocyte is unable to provide efficient ZEBOV reproduction. **Figure 5-6A** shows a dense, irregular-shaped viral inclusion not typical of normal ZEBOV viral inclusions. For example, see Figures 4-3, 5-1, 5-3, and 5-4 for comparison with viral replication of filoviruses in a "normal" hepatocyte. Figure 5-6A also shows budding viral particles (magnification 16,000). **Figure 5-6B** shows the same area at a higher magnification (magnification 38,000).

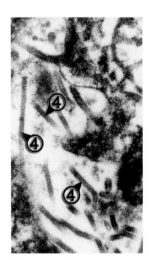

Figure 5-6B

Spleen

We detected filoviral reproduction in the spleen (the largest organ in the lymphatic system), specifically in the splenic red pulp and in the macrophage cells, but only very rarely in the endothelial cells and fibroblasts. The first MARV-infected macrophages in the spleen were found on day 5 following IP inoculation in the sinus lumen and interstitial tissue in monkeys and on day 4 in IP-infected guinea pigs. The first ZEBOV-infected macrophages in the spleen of the monkeys were identified in the sinus lumen on day 3 post-inoculation.

Infected splenic macrophages in all the animals were mature and large and contained multiple phagosomes. The numbers of the infected macrophages did not significantly increase during the course of the filoviral infection. At the terminal stages of the disease, most infected macrophages were destroyed, and the number of "newly" infected macrophages (i.e., macrophages with only limited filoviral infection) was very small. Probably, the spleen contains a limited number of macrophages capable of supporting reproduction of filoviruses. Even at the terminal stage, uninfected macrophages were found in the spleen. These observations may be explained by the different abilities of the macrophage subtypes to support filoviral reproduction. It appears that the spleen has several different macrophage subtypes and only some of them become infected. In contrast, following large infectious doses, all the hepatocytes in filovirus-inoculated animals were found to be infected.

Kidneys

ZEBOV and MARV do not reproduce in the epithelial cells of the kidneys. At the terminal stages of disease, we found rare instances of filoviral reproduction in the kidneys, circulating and interstitial macrophages, single fibroblasts, and endothelial cells. In general, infected cells were extremely rare findings in the kidney sections in all the studied animals.

Lungs

Filoviral hemorrhagic fevers are not associated with marked respiratory symptoms and, for this reason, little attention has been given to the lungs in experimental studies. However, the possible role of lungs in filoviral transmission among humans and animals deserves some consideration because if aerosol transmission is possible, the filoviral diseases may be able to spread readily from human to human.

Role of Lungs in Filovirus Transmission. Several researchers have shown that guinea pigs and monkeys can be infected experimentally with filoviral aerosols [Johnson, 1995; Lub, 1995; Ryabchikova, 1996]; however, direct aerosol transmission of the filoviruses from one animal to another has not been established. Indeed, in the viral diseases where aerosol transmission plays a dominant role, the lungs contain large amounts of the virus and intensive coughing or sneezing is required to release the virus into the air.

Filoviral Reproduction in Lungs. Examination of the lungs in EBOV- and MARV-infected rhesus monkeys has not shown any signs of viral reproduction in the epithelium of bronchi and alveoli, even at the terminal stages of disease [Baskerville, 1985; Johnson, 1995; Murphy, 1971]. Some cells of type II epithelium of the alveoli and bronchi in rhesus monkeys have been reported as capable of supporting REBOV reproduction in cynomolgus monkeys [Geisbert, 1992]. In our time course studies of the lungs in IP-inoculated monkeys and guinea pigs, we observed the reproduction of MARV and ZEBOV in circulating and interstitial macrophages, and infrequently in endothelial cells and fibroblasts. Figure 5-7 shows a ZEBOV-infected circulating macrophage from the lung of a green monkey. These macrophages in the lungs became involved in filoviral reproduction only at the terminal stages of disease.

In aerosol-infected guinea pigs, MARV reproduction in lung sections has also been found in circulating and interstitial macrophages, in alveolar macrophages, but rarely in fibroblasts and endothelial cells even at the late stages of disease. These findings support our conclusion that the mode of infection does not alter the target cells. However, there were a few exceptions in the case of monkey species inoculated with ZEBOV. In these exceptions, alveolar and bronchial cells were infected and showed all the signs of viral reproduction, including formation of viral

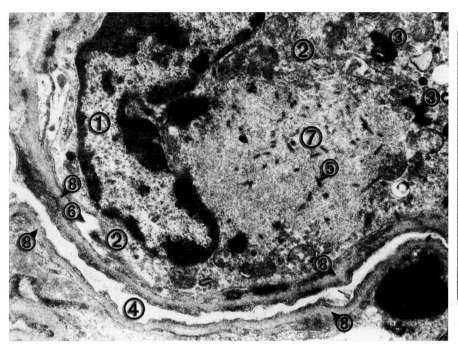

Legend

Figure 5-7

1. Nucleus of macrophage
2. Cytoplasm
3. Phagosome
4. Alveolar space
5. Viral nucleocapsid
6. Capillary lumen
7. Viral inclusion body
8. Basal membrane

See Note on page xiii.

Figure 5-7. An ultrathin section of a green monkey's lung showing replication of ZEBOV in a circulating macrophage (magnification 17,000). The macrophage is located in an alveolar capillary, which has a common basal membrane with the alveole. A viral inclusion body and individual viral particles can be seen. This picture shows that filovirus-infected macrophages may be found in any blood vessel in any organ of the infected animal. (Photo by Dr. L. Kolesnikova)

particles. In Figure 4-7, ZEBOV nucleocapsids and virions (evidence of virus replication) can be seen in the alveolar epithelial cell and in the ciliated cells. The infected epithelial cells were located in those areas of the lungs showing severe damage to lung tissue (i.e., edema, prominent hemorrhages, and leukocytes in alveoli, capillaries, and interstitial tissue). The subsequent changes in permeability may permit the passage of ZEBOV from the blood to the epithelial cells of the alveoli and bronchi and thereby expose them to infection. Viewed broadly, the results of studies on filoviral reproduction in the lungs of monkeys and guinea pigs suggest that the probability for aerosol transmission of the filoviruses between the animals is low. However, the fact that filoviral reproduction can occur in the epithelial cells of the respiratory lining calls for attention to this organ. If the virus changes phenotypically under ecological or experimental influences and initiates competent infections in monkey or human respiratory tracts, filoviruses could become very contagious and extremely dangerous.

Adrenals

The adrenal glands rank after the liver as organs whose parenchymal cells are capable of reproducing the filoviruses. MARV and ZEBOV reproduction (the presence of viral inclusion bodies, viral particles, and nucleocapsids) was observed in adrenal cortical cells of the green monkey. Some of these features can be seen in Figure 4-4, an EM from a ZEBOV-infected green monkey. As in hepatocytes, infection with ZEBOV produces large viral inclusions, while MARV produces small and irregular-shaped inclusion bodies. Numerous viral particles were observed in the intercellular spaces. We also noted filoviral reproduction in the interstitial and circulating macrophages but rarely in fibroblasts and endothelial cells. The other types of adrenal parenchymal cells in monkeys did not support viral reproduction. In guinea pig adrenals, MARV also infected adrenal cortical cells, macrophages, and fibroblasts.

Heart

MARV and ZEBOV do not reproduce in heart muscle cells. Figure 5-8 shows viral replication in a macrophage found in the interstitial tissue of the heart muscle. Only the interstitial macrophages, fibroblasts, and endothelial cells were found to be infected in heart tissue and only at the terminal stages of the disease.

Digestive Tract

The epithelial cells of the stomach, intestines, salivary glands, and pancreas do not support to any extent MARV and ZEBOV reproduction in guinea pigs and monkeys. Filoviral reproduction in these organs was observed only in the interstitial tissue of the lamina propria (the connective tissue beneath the epithelium of these organs) and only in the late stages of the disease. Viral inclusion bodies, nucleocapsids, and virions were discovered in rare fibroblasts and interstitial macrophages.

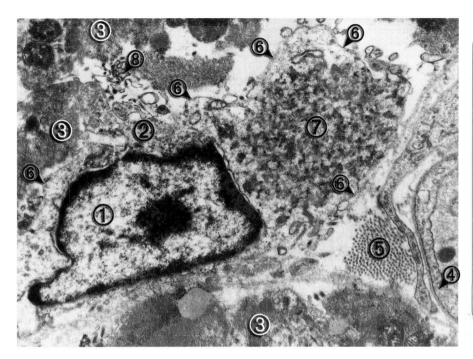

Legend

Figure 5-8

1. Nucleus
2. Cytoplasm
3. Muscle cell
4. Capillary
5. Collagen
6. Macrophage plasma membrane
7. Viral inclusion body
8. Net-like structure

See Note on page xiii.

Figure 5-8. An ultrathin section of the heart of a green monkey infected with ZEBOV shows replication in a macrophage located in interstitial tissue (magnification 12,500). This picture represents another example of how the infected macrophages cause organs and tissues to become infected. This macrophage came to the interstitial tissue of heart muscle and produced viral particles, which in turn may infect the neighboring fibroblasts.

Summary of Target Cells and Target Organs

EBOV and MARV are able to infect various types of cells in monkeys and guinea pigs. Without question, the first and most important cell in the infection is the macrophage. Macrophages enable the filoviruses to accumulate in blood and thereby disseminate the filoviruses throughout the organisms. Infected macrophages, joined later by infected fibroblasts and endothelial cells, eventually infected all organs. We were able to show the initial filoviral infection of macrophages and subsequent progress of infections in cells and organs over the time of the disease development. This process is shown in the schematic presented in Figure 5-9. The circulating and resident macrophages are the target cells. The hepatocytes, adrenal cortical cells, splenic macrophages, interstitial macrophages, endothelial cells, and

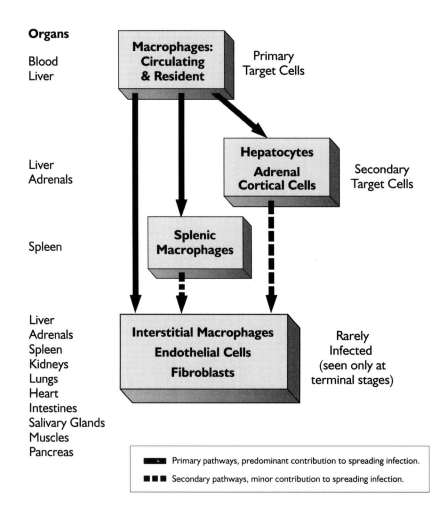

Figure 5-9. The schematic depicts the progression of ZEBOV and MARV infection of tissues and organs in fatally infected monkeys and guinea pigs. The primary target cell is the macrophage. The infected macrophages release virions, which circulate in the blood and lymph systems. These are carried along to other organs, where they infect liver and adrenal parenchyma (i.e., the hepatocytes in the liver and the adrenal cortex cells of the adrenals). The macrophages in every organ are eventually infected. The last cells to be infected are the endothelial cells in the spleen, lungs, kidneys, and other organs.

fibroblasts are all secondary target cells. Although endothelial cells and tissues do become infected, they do so only at the terminal stages of the disease and so are not target cells.

The macrophages are infected and release virions (or virus progeny), which in turn infect more macrophages, hepatocytes (liver parenchyma), adrenal cortical cells (adrenal parenchyma), and eventually fibroblasts and endothelial cells in the liver, adrenals, spleen, kidneys, lungs, and other tissues. Even though filoviral infection occurs in parenchymal tissues, these infections are not critical to the disease process. The pathology of the circulation system was not discussed in this chapter but it is crucial to understanding the disease. Because of its importance, the blood system is discussed separately in the following chapter.

chapter 6

Blood Disorders in Filoviral Infections

Various clinical descriptions of MARV and EBOV infections describe subcutaneous bleeding and bleeding from the mouth, eyes, and ears as one of the most notable signs and symptoms of these diseases. Indeed, "hemorrhages from all the body's orifices" is one of the most vivid descriptions in *The Hot Zone* [Preston, 1994]. Although infected humans rarely die from blood loss, the term "hemorrhagic fever" connotes the severe damage to blood vessels seen in filovirus-infected humans and animals. The source of the hemorrhages and their significance in the development of fatal Ebola and Marburg diseases are crucial questions in understanding the pathology of the infections. In this chapter, we analyze the disorders that develop in the blood system in experimental animals and explore their significance and relationships in the development of Marburg and Ebola viral diseases.

Clinical Manifestations

Clinical observations provide the evidence for profound disturbances in the clotting mechanism and in vessel permeability in patients with Marburg and Ebola diseases.

Disseminated intravascular coagulation (DIC) has been observed in Ebola hemorrhagic fever and has been noted in cases of Marburg fever [Cosgriff, 1989]. DIC reflects an imbalance between the clot promoting and lysing systems.

Hemorrhage is the most impressive and severe of the clinical symptoms of filoviral hemorrhagic fevers. However, not every filovirus-infected human exhibits hemorrhages. Large individual variations exist in the degree and characteristics and therefore signs of damage to the blood system. According to LeGuenno, this severe symptom develops in 60% of Ebola fever human cases [LeGuenno, 1997]. The appearance of hemorrhages usually signals a turn for the worse in the course of the disease; however, the disease also may be fatal without visible hemorrhages. The most gripping events in EBOV-infected monkeys include sporadic bleeding from the injection site, vomiting blood, bleeding from the rectum and vagina, and hemorrhaging of the skin and mucous membranes. As in humans, pronounced individual variability was noted in the extent and type of blood alterations in filovirus-infected monkeys [Fisher-Hoch, 1992; Johnson, 1995]. Only 40-45% of ZEBOV-infected baboons showed this hemorrhage syndrome [Luchko, 1995]. The exact mechanism of hemorrhage development in humans and in monkeys remains unclear.

The risk of hemorrhage restricts blood sampling and other invasive procedures in humans. These precautions often preclude the continuous monitoring required to adequately evaluate filoviral damage to the blood system. Both in hospitals and in research laboratories, investigators take precautions to avoid exposure to the hazardous filoviruses. This fear of infection provides one reason for the emotional visual observations describing DIC and hemorrhagic syndromes, such as those noted in *The Hot Zone* and *Outbreak*. Some of this fear is misplaced and may also occur as a result of limited medical knowledge. For example, natural outbreaks of Ebola hemorrhagic fever have occurred in African villages. But it is the remoteness of the villages, lack of medical services, and fear of infection that contribute to the scarcity of published data with respect to damage and the condition of the blood systems in filovirus-infected humans.

Blood-clotting inability was also noted in animals that succumbed to MARV disease in the earliest experiments [Siegert,

1967; Siegert, 1968; Zlotnik, 1969]. Visible hemorrhages were not observed in rhesus monkeys at the terminal stages of MARV infection, although the blood clotting time increased from 2 min 42 sec to 85 min, and fibrinogen was absent from their blood [Lub, 1995]. Signs of profound perturbation to the blood clotting system were also observed in rhesus monkeys infected with large doses of EBOV. The levels of clotting factors (I, VII, and VIII) were decreased and thromboplastin and prothrombin times were increased [Fisher-Hoch, 1985]. In some of the EBOV-infected rhesus monkeys, fibrin degradation products were seen before death, indicating DIC had developed [Fisher-Hoch, 1985; Jaax, 1996]. Our studies of ZEBOV infection in baboons revealed the development of DIC, which was characterized by a very short period of hypercoagulation and followed by an abnormally long period of hypocoagulation. These baboons bled from the rectum and nose and exhibited hemorrhages in skin and mucous membranes [Luchko, 1995; Ryabchikova, 1999a]. Published data on the pathophysiology of the blood system in filovirus-infected humans and animals are very fragmentary and inadequate to support definite conclusions about the mechanisms of the blood system damage caused by EBOV and MARV.

Morphologic Observations

Few studies have described the damage to blood vessels in EBOV- and MARV-infected animals at the microscopic level. This is likely because applications of large infectious doses of the viruses result in high degrees of lesions, which mask details. However, descriptions of the pathological changes in the blood system of filovirus-infected animals have been published. The pathological changes noted at the terminal stages of Ebola disease in monkeys include destruction of the endothelial layer in hepatic sinusoids, splenic sinuses, and renal parenchyma capillaries. Numerous fibrin thrombi in the small blood vessels, and hemorrhages caused by erythrocyte diapedesis into the visceral organs, while common findings in all filoviral diseases, were more prominent in EBOV infections [Baskerville, 1978; Jaax, 1996; Johnson, 1995, Peters, 1996].

Microscopic study alone cannot provide a comprehensive set of facts and explanations about the blood system's changes. Microscopic examination can capture the state of the organs at a definite moment (i.e., a photograph). Comparison of these photographs, showing different objects in the same circumstances, may provide additional information leading to an analysis of the circumstances. For our studies, we used various doses of ZEBOV and MARV and, as described in Chapter 5, examined samples daily from the animals. Using this strategy, we could examine even apparently isolated events of blood system damage and analyze their significance and contribution to filoviral pathogenicity. We used microscopy to compare the alterations in the blood systems and to help clarify the development of blood disorders in Ebola and Marburg diseases.

Time Course of Pathomorphological Changes in the Blood System

The common feature of Ebola and Marburg disease in all the studied animals was severe changes in the microcirculation system (capillaries, postcapillary veins, arterioles, small veins, and arteries). The time course studies revealed that the pathological changes in all the infected guinea pigs and monkeys followed a very similar pattern. However, monkeys exhibited more pronounced damage compared to guinea pigs at the same stage of Marburg disease (identical infectious doses were administered). Furthermore, the vascular changes in green monkeys infected with ZEBOV appeared more severe than those infected with MARV. Guinea pigs infected with non-adapted ZEBOV did not die and only their hepatic monocytes and macrophages were infected. However, hepatic inflammation was observed.

The pattern of changes in blood microvessels was similar in all examined organs but varied in degree. Organs having a well-developed vasculature and a good blood supply, namely the liver, spleen, lungs, and kidneys, were the most severely impaired. In these organs, changes in the blood vessels were evident from days 2 and 3 post-inoculation in all the animals infected with ZEBOV and MARV. Figure 6-1 shows some of the changes in the blood circulation in the liver, kidneys, and lungs of ZEBOV-infected monkeys. We observed stasis in capillaries, venules and small

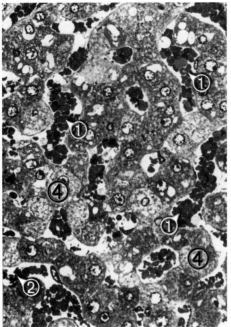

Figure 6-1A

Figure 6-1B

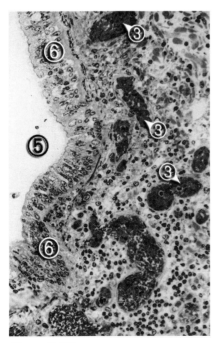

Figure 6-1C

Figure 6-1. Light microscope photographs showing changes in the blood circulation in the liver, kidney, and lung tissues in ZEBOV-infected monkeys. These photographs show widespread changes in microcirculation. Agglutinated erythrocytes forming small thrombi are visible in the blood vessels in all these photographs. These changes are identical regardless of whether the filovirus has infected the parenchyma cells. In **Figure 6-1A**, the liver tissue shows no evidence of inflammation (i.e., no leukocytes or accumulations of leukocytes). In **Figure 6-1B**, although the renal epithelium is unable to replicate filoviruses, prominent microcirculatory disturbances are obvious as seen by the erythrocyte thrombi. **Figure 6-1C** shows the agglutinated erythrocytes.

Legend

Figure 6-1

1. Erythrocyte thrombi

2. Rouleaux

3. Clogged capillary and small vessel

4. Hepatocyte

5. Bronchi lumen

6. Bronchi epithelium

7. Renal glomerulus

8. Renal canaliculi

See Note on page xiii.

veins, erythrocyte sludge and rouleaux (cylindrical masses of erythrocytes), and erythrocyte thrombi. We also observed a marked
decrease in endothelial pinocytosis (uptake of fluids into endothelial cells) and an engorgement of the small veins and venules by
blood cells. Small thrombi composed of platelets and single blood
cells were occasionally observed. In the other organs (i.e., those
with less developed vasculature), we found fewer changes within
the first 5 days of the infection, and the endothelial cells were
unchanged. Thus, it appears that microcirculation was altered
from the very early stages of the infection. As a result of the
changed circulation, oxygen deprivation of tissues occurred in
filovirus-infected animals. Other researchers were able to associ-
ate the thrombi in the gut of infected monkeys with increased
endotoxin, a factor in shock and another aspect of the pathogenesis [Jaax, 1996].

Disturbances of microvasculature in all organs become more
pronounced as the disease develops. The increase in damage was
more marked in the liver, spleen, kidneys, and lungs than in the
heart, intestines, pancreas, and salivary glands. At the terminal
stages of filoviral infection, in the liver, spleen, lungs, and kidneys,
the microvasculature showed severely impaired structure and
blood flow. Erythrocytes, fibrin, swollen neutrophils, and cell
debris obstructed the lumens of the vessels in these organs.
Figure 6-1 shows capillaries and small vessels clogged with erythrocytes in a ZEBOV-infected monkey. Figure 6-2 shows fibrin
thrombi in the blood vessels of the adrenal gland and lung in
ZEBOV-infected monkeys.

Figure 6-2. Two different views of microcirculation damage
in tissues. **Figure 6-2A** shows a light microscope photograph
of a semithin section of an adrenal gland of a rhesus monkey
infected with ZEBOV. Also notable in this photograph is the
absence of an inflammatory reaction to infected adrenal cells.
Figure 6-2B shows an electron microscope photograph of
fibrin thrombi in blood vessels in the interstitial lung tissue of
a green monkey infected by ZEBOV (magnification 9,500).
Two kinds of fibrin deposits can be seen. The left vessel is
tightly clogged by fibrin, but the right vessel contains a
crumbly fibrin deposit.

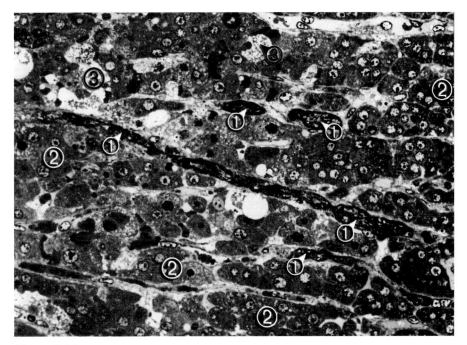

Figure 6-2A

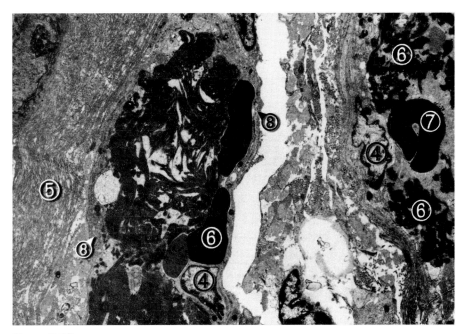

Figure 6-2B

Legend

Figure 6-2

1. Fibrin thrombi
2. Adrenal gland cell
3. Necroses
4. Endothelial cell
5. Interstitial tissue
6. Fibrin
7. Erythrocyte
8. Blood vessel wall

See Note on page xiii.

Figure 6-3 shows the accumulation of neutrophils in an alveo-lar capillary of a ZEBOV-infected monkey, along with probable blood vessel wall damage. These changes to the microvasculature occur even when the parenchyma cells are not infected and are often accompanied by other changes visible in the tissues.

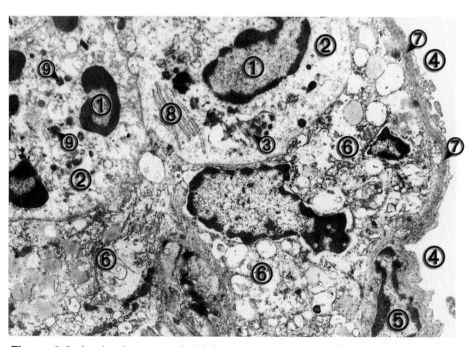

Legend

Figure 6-3

1. Nucleus of neutrophil

2. Cytoplasm

3. Phagosome

4. Alveolar space

5. Endothelial cell

6. Alveolar cell

7. Basal membrane

8. Endoplasmic reticulum (ER) in neutrophil cytoplasm

9. Lysosome

See Note on page xiii.

Figure 6-3. An ultrathin section highlighting the accumulation of neutrophils in an alveolar capillary in a ZEBOV-infected green monkey (magnification 7,000). The presence of neutrophils in the lung's capillary bed indicates not only blockage, but also probable damage to blood vessel walls. Neutrophils release proteolytic enzymes and active oxygen intermediators. The proteolytic enzymes and the active oxygen intermediators damage cell membranes and blood vessel walls.

Endothelial cells often were swollen and many became necrotic. Figure 6-4 shows the destroyed endothelial cells in an arteriole in the spleen of a ZEBOV-infected monkey. Not all kinds of vessels were altered to the same degree, even in the liver and spleen. The most severe lesions were observed at the post-capillary venules, where molecular and cellular exchange between blood and tissue occurs; however, the arterioles were not markedly altered. Note that despite the extensive infections, numerous endothelial cells remained morphologically unaltered in the heart, intestines, lymphatic tissue, pancreas, and salivary glands, even up to death of the animals. These cells were not infected by the filoviruses and were generally unaffected by other influences of the infection's progression.

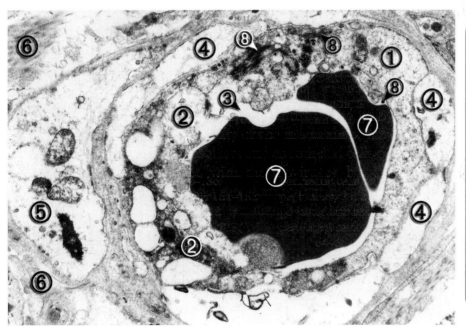

Legend

Figure 6-4

1. Endothelial cell
2. Destroyed endothelial cell
3. Arteriole lumen
4. Swollen muscle cell
5. Podocyte
6. Interstitial tissue
7. Erythrocyte
8. Viral nucleocapsid

See Note on page xiii.

Figure 6-4. A small arteriole in the spleen of a rhesus monkey infected with ZEBOV (magnification 10,000). This photograph shows the high degree of vessel lesions. All components of the vessel wall are altered. There are obvious lesions in both endothelial and smooth muscle cells. Even so, not all the endothelial cells are affected.

Figure 6-5 shows that fibrin deposition occurred in the intestines, an organ that does not support ZEBOV replication, and that the endothelial cells did not contain visible lesions.

Legend

Figure 6-5

1. Endothelial cell
2. Fibrin bundle
3. Erythrocyte
4. Interstitial tissue
5. Lumen of vein
6. Basal membrane

See Note on page xiii.

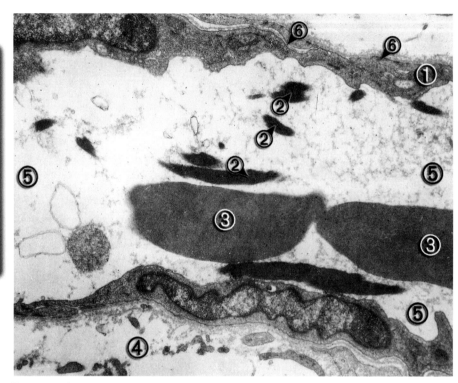

Figure 6-5A

Figure 6-5B

Figure 6-5. Epithelial cells in intestines are not infected even at the terminal stages of filoviral disease. **Figure 6-5A** illustrates two items: fibrin deposits in the vessel of an organ not supporting ZEBOV replication, and absence of lesions in the endothelial cells (magnification 11,000). The unaltered endothelial cells of a small vein in the large intestine of a green monkey infected with ZEBOV are visible. A view of a fibrin fiber at higher magnification is shown in **Figure 6-5B** (magnification 100,000). Note the characteristic striations of the fibrin fiber.

Since we found that the endothelium and muscle walls in medium-sized arteries and veins were unchanged, we concentrated our examinations on the microcirculation system. We found no damage in the medium-sized vessels, so we did not examine the main blood vessels. The most extensive damage observed was to the terminal chains in the blood system (i.e., the post-capillary venules and capillaries); this damage plays a significant role in the development of Ebola and Marburg diseases in filovirus-infected animals.

Other changes in the blood system morphology that are evident are hemorrhages and clotting. Multiple hemorrhages are evidence of hypocoagulation and damage to the permeability of blood vessels. Hypercoagulation, the presence of fibrin clots, bundles, and thrombi, are the morphological evidence of DIC. Both DIC and hemorrhagic syndromes are complicated pathophysiological events regulated by a complex balance of various biologically active substances (e.g., clotting and other factors). In clinical practice, microscopic examinations can be used to confirm the diagnosis of DIC in autopsies. The exact biochemical parameters related to the morphological observations are not well known. Some researchers consider that DIC occurs only under the condition that fibrin thrombi and depositions are abundant at postmortem examination [Hamilton, 1978]. We use the notation of "morphological signs of DIC" to describe the microscopic observations of multiple fibrin deposits and thrombi found through all the examined organs.

Our studies did not reveal morphological signs of DIC in monkeys and guinea pigs infected with MARV by various routes and doses. Our organ sections from these animals showed fibrin deposition only in the necrotic areas, where fibrin masses in necrotic tissues were produced by plasma exudate. This feature of fibrin deposition needs to be considered during histopathological examinations of organs when diagnosing DIC. Some green monkeys showed slight erythrocyte diapedesis in the spleen and liver, without the formation of conspicuous hemorrhages. These observations are in agreement with known clinical manifestations of Marburg disease in monkeys and guinea pigs.

ZEBOV caused more variations in blood damage in monkeys (as compared with other species and MARV). In some monkeys, fibrin deposits and clots were found, while in other species, hemorrhages were more common. Examinations of the late stages of ZEBOV infection in green and rhesus monkeys showed numerous fibrin thrombi and fibrin bundles in blood vessels, morphological signs of DIC. These fibrin bodies can be seen in Figures 6-5A and 6-5B, sections from the intestines of a ZEBOV-infected green monkey. Fibrin thrombi on the surface of a macrophage from a green monkey liver are apparent in Figure 6-6. Fibrin clots were observed in all the organs we studied, even in those whose tissues poorly supported viral growth such as the intestines, salivary glands, and heart muscles. However, we did not see fibrin thrombi in the organs from baboons in the terminal stages of Ebola disease. In Figure 6-7 (light and electron microscope photographs of baboon adrenal glands), numerous hemorrhages are apparent.

Legend

Figure 6-6

1. Nucleus of macrophage

2. Lumen of hepatic sinusoid

3. Erythrocyte

4. Destroyed cell

5. Phagosome in macrophage

6. Fibrin clot

See Note on page xiii.

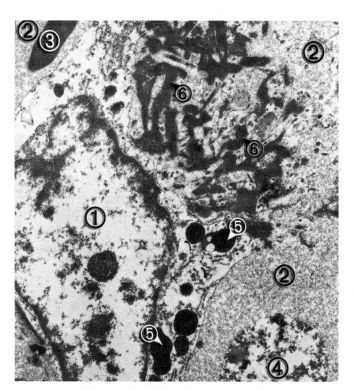

Figure 6-6. The relation of fibrin clots to the surface of a macrophage in a green monkey liver. Macrophages play a significant role in the alteration of the blood system by producing and releasing biologically active substances (cytokines) (magnification 8,000).

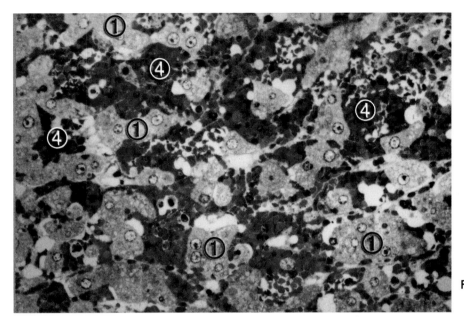

See Note on page xiii.

Legend

Figure 6-7

1. Adrenal cell
2. Interstitial tissue
3. Macrophage
4. Erythrocyte

Figure 6-7A

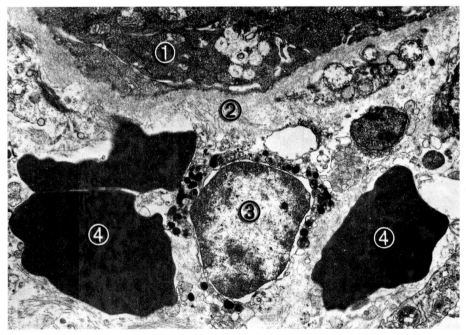

Figure 6-7B

Figure 6-7. Light and electron microscope pictures of ZEBOV-infected baboon adrenal gland tissue that demonstrates prominent hemorrhages. **Figure 6-7A** (the light microscope photograph) shows the prominence of hemorrhages. **Figure 6-7B** (the electron microscope photograph), the hemorrhage is seen as erythrocytes lying outside the vessels in the interstitial tissue (magnification 7,000). (Photos by Dr. L. Kolesnikova)

Hemorrhages could be seen in the baboons' visceral organs in the days before death. This is consistent with the blood chemistry data showing blood hypocoagulation during the same time period of ZEBOV infection.

Thus, damage to the blood system in monkeys infected with ZEBOV represents a combination of microcirculatory disturbances, fibrin deposition, and hemorrhage. Hemostasis and erythrocyte aggregation impairing the blood supply were noted in the capillaries and small vessels of the visceral organs in all monkey species. However, we noted that the morphological picture of blood vessel damage looked different in four monkey species (baboons, rhesus, cynomolgus, and green monkeys), and so we performed an experiment comparing the pathologies of these monkey species to examine the species differences.

Species-Related Differences in EBOV-Infected Monkeys

Monkey species differ in their sensitivity to filoviruses and in their clinical manifestations [Fisher-Hoch, 1992; Ryabchikova, 1998; Ryabchikova, 1999a]. Our studies showed that baboons are less susceptible to equivalent doses of ZEBOV when compared to African green and rhesus monkeys, and baboons more frequently have hemorrhages. Cynomolgus monkeys did not develop signs of DIC and the course of disease was protracted. They usually died 10–14 days after inoculation, baboons died 9–10 days after inoculation, and rhesus and green monkeys died 7–8 days after inoculation. Other researchers have noted that their cynomolgus monkeys died 7–8 days after inoculation with ZEBOV [Jahrling, 1999; Geisbert, 2002]. Some of the parameters that may give different results are the different infectious dose, the age and source of the monkeys, as well as the difference in the source of and the processing of the virus. The research done at USAMRIID notes that ZEBOV isolated from a human patient in 1995 was used. The ZEBOV used at Vector (described in Chapter 2) was from the 1976 outbreak in Zaire.

We decided to compare pathological changes in the blood vessels in these four monkey species. All monkey species received identical small doses of ZEBOV (1–10 LD_{50} for corresponding species) and their organs were sampled for microscopic examination at the terminal stages of the disease. Species-specific differences of blood system damage in ZEBOV-infected monkeys were observed in more than 30 animals. These data are not coincidences but are a sign that differences exist in the mechanisms damaging the blood systems. A summary of the results for this series is presented in Table 6-1. It is noted that for all the species in Table 6-1, blood cell counts showed an increase in neutrophils and a decrease in lymphocytes and platelets.

There was damage to the microcirculation system in the four monkey species, but the pattern was different in each. The pattern of vascular lesions appeared identical in green and rhesus monkeys. This pattern is visible in Figures 6-2, 6-5, and 6-6. The blood vessels contain multiple fibrin thrombi and bundles, and fibrin depositions are also found around the vessels. The pattern of blood vessel damage in these species is evidence that at the terminal stages of Ebola disease, the hypercoagulation stage of DIC had developed.

Table 6-1. Species-specific characteristics of ZEBOV-infected monkeys.*

Species	Time to Death	Blood Condition
Green monkeys	7–8 d	Fibrin clots
Rhesus monkeys	7–8 d	Fibrin clots
Cynomolgus monkeys	10–14 d	No hemorrhage, no clot Capillary stasis Erythrocyte aggregation Organs engorged with blood
Baboons	9–10 d	Erythrocyte diapedisis

* Dose, 1–10 LD_{50}, SC inoculation

Cynomolgus monkeys showed signs of prominent capillary stasis, erythrocyte aggregation, and engorgement with blood cells, indicating damage to the blood supply of organs and tissues. We did not observe any morphologic evidence of clotting or hemorrhages in the blood tissues of these monkeys, despite the high level of ZEBOV reproduction.

Examination of the baboon tissues revealed a third type of blood system damage at the terminal stages of Ebola disease. These tissues showed prominent hemorrhages and erythrocyte diapedesis, indicative of the development of the hemorrhagic syndrome and characteristic of vascular damage. This is seen in Figures 6-7A and 6-7B, where these hemorrhages are visible in the blood vessels from the adrenal glands. Examination of the hemorrhagic areas in the skin and visceral organs in these baboons showed that the hemorrhages are not associated with destruction or inflammation of the vessel walls. They form by diapedesis of erythrocytes (i.e., the erythrocytes migrate between structurally unaltered endothelial cells) (Figure 6-8). The erythrocytes are localized outside the vessels and no changes to their structures were observed over the last 2 days before death. We did not find a relationship between the sites of hemorrhage and filovirus-infected endothelial or macrophage cells. This implies that infected macrophages and endothelial cells are not directly responsible for the erythrocytes' exit from the blood vessels. In other words, erythrocytes do not use the infected cells as a gate for the exit from blood vessels. Rather, the factors inducing hemorrhage come from the bloodstream (i.e., they are humoral). We believe that macrophage mediators (i.e., cytokines released by the macrophage) play a leading role in inducing these hemorrhages. Neutrophils take part in tissue and vessel injury by mediator release [Fujishima, 1995; Janoff, 1982] and pericytes may also contribute to hemorrhage development. We detected swelling of the pericytes and smooth muscle cells in the wall of vessels located in the hemorrhagic zones. Pericytes are known to regulate vessel permeability [Lonigro, 1996], so their damage in filovirus-infected animals may also be important for hemorrhage development.

Our observations, combined with other published research, lead us to conclude that microcirculatory disturbances leading to alteration of blood supply of organs are common and are the most sig-

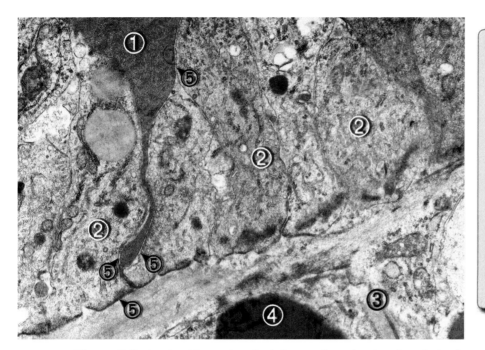

Legend

Figure 6-8

1. Erythrocyte moving across endothelial layer
2. Endothelial cell
3. Interstitial tissue
4. Erythrocyte in the interstitial tissue
5. Plasma membrane of endothelial cell

See Note on page xiii.

Figure 6-8. An ultrathin section of a baboon spleen showing diapedesis of erythrocytes into interstitial tissue (magnification 14,000). Diapedesis is an active movement of blood cells outside the vessel, through undamaged wall. This is the normal movement for leukocytes to enter tissues to carry out their functions. Diapedesis of erythrocytes (erythrodiapedesis) is a characteristic of the pathology of the hemorrhages in ZEBOV infections.

nificant pathogenic link in all EBOV- and MARV-infected animals. Other clinical manifestations, even those severe disturbances such as hemorrhages and fibrin thrombosis, appear to be dependent on the individual infected animal species and may not be necessarily linked to lethality.

Possible Mechanisms

Our examination and analysis of the blood system pathology in animals infected with MARV and ZEBOV identified the events common to all animals, those common to different species, and the variations within the same animal species. Understanding of the possible causes of the different manifestations of damage (microcirculatory disturbances, hemorrhages, and clotting) to the blood system, and the role of the various blood cell types (macrophages, neutrophils, lymphocytes, platelets, and endothelial cells) in producing the damage, is critical to a more complete understanding of the diseases.

One attractive idea is to link the filoviral replication in endothelial cells with damage to the blood system. However, our studies and others have shown that damage to the endothelial cells is not caused directly by viral infections. Pathological changes to endothelial cells usually developed independently of filoviral replication and began to appear from 3 to 4 days post-inoculation, depending on the infectious dose, despite the fact that viral replication in endothelial cells was not observed until late in the disease, if at all. Similar data were reported by other researchers who looked at ZEBOV (strain Mayinga) infections in guinea pigs and also concluded that endothelial cell infection and fibrin deposition occurred later in the disease [Connolly, 1999].

The hemorrhages and clotting characteristics of some of the diseases appear to result from the development of DIC. DIC may develop in the course of numerous diseases and clinical conditions, even without any infectious agent, so identifying all the factors that could induce DIC would be very complicated. DIC may develop as a result of activation of the blood monocytes, the primary sources of the thromboplastin needed to transform fibrinogen into fibrin. Researchers have shown that damaged endothelial cells are involved in the development of DIC, but to a lesser extent than activation of blood monocytes [Ratnoff, 1984]. It is very tempting to suggest that the infection of the monocytes (or macrophages) with EBOV gives rise directly to DIC. However, although the macrophages are the primary targets for filoviral infections in all the animals, not every animal develops DIC. We suggest that ZEBOV-infected macrophages (perhaps stimulated during filoviral infection) trigger the release of thromboplastin from the monocytes or macrophages. It is possible that only some of the filoviral proteins, and not the entire virus, could be involved in this triggering.

We did not observe DIC in MARV disease of either monkeys or guinea pigs, but we did observe this in monkeys infected with ZEBOV. One main difference between MARV and EBOV is that EBOV has a non-structural glycoprotein, the small, secreted glycoprotein (sGP). Other researchers have reported that EBOV replication is associated with synthesis and secretion of large amounts of sGP [Volchkov, 1995; Volchkov, 1998; Feldmann, 1999]. Perhaps this sGP acts as a direct or indirect trigger, at least in monkeys, to induce DIC. In fact, in our studies, DIC with fibrin thrombosis was not shown to develop in MARV-infected animals. MARV does not produce sGP. We hypothesize that GP1 and/or sGP may bind to the receptors on the monocytes and thereby may induce thromboplastin release and subsequent DIC development. Moreover, it is quite conceivable that the GP1 and sGP may bind differently to the monocytes in different monkey species. This selectivity in binding may be responsible for the observed differences in the pattern of blood disorders in different monkey species infected with EBOV. Using this hypothesis, the sGP or GP1 (or perhaps both) would bind to receptors on the monocytes in green and rhesus monkeys, and in so doing, would induce fibrinogen polymerization and fibrin clots. The nature of binding may be different in baboons; in baboons, the binding may trigger changes in blood vessel permeability and thus result in hemorrhages. In cynomolgus monkeys, GPs may not bind to the monocytes, and consequently, neither DIC nor hemorrhagic syndrome develops. Further, this interaction of the GP molecules with monkey monocytes could be related to expressions of different receptors on the monocyte surface, and these different receptors may be determined genetically and thus be a species-related difference. The interaction of GP molecules with receptors implying a possible genetic link could also extend to differences in human filoviral infections.

Another possibility could be that sGP and GP1 of EBOV act on the macrophage level rather than on the monocytes. The GPs may selectively bind to different macrophage subsets causing the release of different mediators, which in turn may trigger fibrin polymerization or hemorrhage development. This mechanism would explain the species-specific differences between monkeys and also the observed variations in damage to the blood system in EBOV-infected humans, similar to the discussion above. Regardless of how the GPs interact, these compounds require more study before their roles are understood.

Vascular permeability changes are another aspect of the disease in filovirus-infected monkeys. These changes may be triggered by a set of humoral mediators produced from macrophages. *In vitro* studies have shown that the supernatant derived from MARV-infected macrophages alters the permeability of the endothelial layer. The change in permeability was attributed to tumor necrosis factor (TNF), one of the known macrophage mediators [Feldmann, 1996a]. These findings are consistent with our assumption that the macrophage mediators play a leading role in blood disorders.

Although the role of macrophages is pivotal in filoviral infections, neutrophils may also have a role. Neutrophils, among their other functions, interact directly with blood vessel walls and produce many substances influencing vessel permeability [Witko-Sarsat, 2000]. The significance of the neutrophils in altering blood vessel permeability in filoviral diseases needs further investigation. One report suggested that secreted GP interacts and binds with neutrophils [Yang, 1998]; however, more recent research indicates that there is no interaction and that it is "unlikely that sGP plays a role in the Ebola virus pathogenesis through interfering with the innate immunity by targeting neutrophils" [Sui, 2002]. Changes in the blood vessel permeability will involve the endothelial cells and, although these cells are not infected until late in the disease progression, other factors (probably cytokines) released during the infection may affect these cells. Some research, using molecular biological methods and genes expressing ZEBOV GP in adenovirus vectors, has shown that ZEBOV GP altered the endothelial cells *in vitro* and explanted blood vessels from humans and non-human primates in *ex-vivo* cultures [Yang, 2000]. This research may implicate the glycoproteins in the development of hemorrhages, but the exact relationship of this artificial system with natural filoviral infections needs to be elaborated. While both EBOV and MARV have glycoproteins, the glycoproteins have different properties. Based on our observations, the interactions of the glycoproteins in filoviral infections may produce greater damage to the blood system in ZEBOV-infected animals than in MARV infections.

Research, including our own, indicates that a common event in all filovirus-infected animals is damage to the microcirculation system, which leads to the breakdown of oxygen and nutrient supply to all organs. Such severe complications as DIC and hemorrhage syndromes depend on both the viral and animal species and are not a routine pathogenic event during filoviral infection. Development of hemostatic pathology in filovirus-infected animals most probably is related to disturbances in the cytokine profile, which is triggered by infection of monocyte-macrophage cells.

Blood Cell Counts

The filoviruses' effect on the blood system is not limited to microcirculatory damage. They also alter the blood cell composition and numbers, both in monkeys and humans. Other researchers have reported neutrophilia, lymphopenia, and thrombocytopenia in EBOV-infected rhesus and cynomolgus monkeys [Fisher-Hoch, 1985; Fisher-Hoch, 1992; Jaax, 1996; Johnson, 1995; Bray, 2001]. Examination of blood cells in baboons revealed the same changes, with no significant alteration of the erythrocyte number. An interesting finding was the constancy of the relative proportion of T- and B-lymphocytes on a background of progressing lymphopenia [Luchko, 1995]. In the course of MARV disease, the content of lymphocytes decreased in monkeys and guinea pigs [Lub, 1995; Siegert, 1968], but thrombocytopenia and neutropenia were reported only in monkeys [Siegert, 1968]. Filovirus-infected humans and animals show a profound drop in platelet count, which may approach 78–80% [Luchko, 1995; Connolly, 1999; Formenty, 1999; Bray, 2001]. Pronounced lymphopenia is another feature of changes in blood count in humans during Ebola and Marburg hemorrhagic fevers [Peters, 1996; Zaki, 1997; Formenty, 1999]. In studies of ZEBOV-infected humans during the epidemics in Gabon, the blood work showed evidence of massive cellular apoptosis in the blood, which may be a cause of lymphopenia [Baize, 1999].

Although changes in blood cell content are a consistent feature of the clinical picture in filovirus-infected subjects, the mechanisms for these changes remain unknown. Filoviruses do not reproduce in lymphocytes, so lymphopenia must be caused by factors other than direct virus replication. One possibility is that lymphocytes and platelets may be destroyed by the host response to the virus or by the virus' molecular factors during the infection. However, we did not find large bodies of dead blood cells in the visceral organs of filovirus-infected animals. Conversely, some lymphocytes in the lymphatic tissues showed signs of apoptosis during the last 2 days of the disease. While our studies used low doses of ZEBOV, other researchers using high doses of ZEBOV have found evidence of lymphocyte apoptosis in lymphatic organs of infected monkeys [Geisbert, 2000]. Our results are not necessarily contradictory since by using the small doses for the time course study, we would expect to see an increased level of detail for all the events. In any case, it is difficult to count the number of dead cells in tissues and conclude how apoptosis contributed to blood lymphopenia in filoviral diseases. This is an area requiring further studies.

Another possible mechanism to explain lymphopenia and thrombocytopenia may be changes in the production of blood components. We did not study changes in bone marrow during our time course experiments; we examined it only at the terminal stages of ZEBOV and MARV diseases. Our bone marrow samples from all animals contained many infected macrophages. Areas adjacent to infected macrophages were necrotic and contained cellular debris and fibrin depositions, often associated with the macrophage surface. Examination of bone marrow showed occasional necroses of the hemopoietic cells and cells of the sinusoid lining and pronounced damage in the formation of lymphocytes in filovirus-infected animals. While numerous neutrophils and erythrocytes at various stages of formation and maturation were present in the bone marrow, cells indicating formation of monocytes and lymphocytes were extremely rare. Platelets did not form on the surface of the megakaryocytes or the platelets on the surface were devoid of specific granules. This can be seen in Figure 6-9, a bone marrow tissue sample from a MARV-infected guinea pig. Without specific granules, the platelets formed by the megakaryocytes are functionally incompetent. Other researchers have shown that platelets are unable to aggregate in EBOV-infected rhesus monkeys [Fisher-Hoch, 1985]. Some of the megakaryocytes in our studies appear unaltered, while others show pathological changes of varying degrees up to cell necrosis. These pronounced pathological changes might be responsible for producing changes in blood cell counts characteristic of filoviral diseases. The pattern of changes we observed in hemopoiesis agrees well with the changes we noted in blood cell counts in filovirus-infected experimental animals [Luchko, 1995].

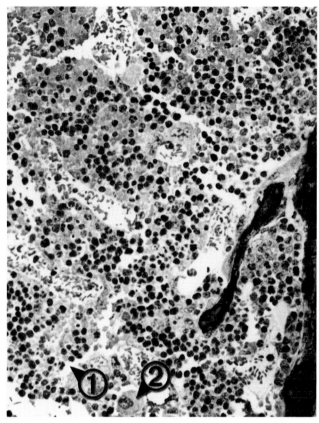

Figure 6-9A

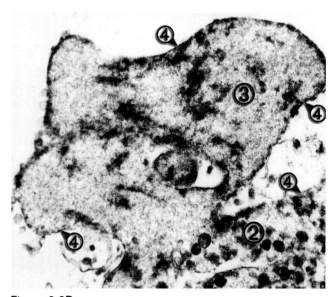

Figure 6-9B

Legend

Figure 6-9

1. Sinus

2. Megakaryocyte

3. Platelet cytoplasm

4. Platelet plasma membrane

See Note on page xiii.

Figure 6-9. The bone marrow tissue from a MARV-infected guinea pig. **Figure 6-9A** shows the semithin section of bone marrow tissue from a guinea pig infected with MARV. The bone marrow is the main organ responsible for producing new blood cells. Damage of the bone marrow causes changes in the entire blood system. This figure also shows that there is no mitosis in the hemopoietic tissue. **Figure 6-9B** shows that there is no evidence of granules in the newly formed platelets from the megakaryocyte (magnification 24,000). Without granules, platelets cannot function and will not aggregate.

The lack of signs of filoviral reproduction in hemopoietic cells suggests that humoral agents cause the hemopoietic derangement. We believe macrophage cells play a role in this. Normal bone marrow hemopoiesis makes the largest contributions to the cellular microenvironment [Akira, 1993; Bogdan, 1993; Campbell, 1988]. Macrophages are components of this microenvironment, and so their destruction itself can result in damage of the hemopoietic tissue. Moreover, filoviral infection of the macrophages may lead to release of the mediators, which can affect hemopoietic tissue. Macrophage mediators, cytokines, interfere with hemopoiesis [Cook, 1996; Sato, 1995]. Additionally, the influence of filoviral proteins liberated from the infected cells cannot be ruled out.

Conclusion

We have used our electron microscope studies to examine the roles and causes of blood disorders in filoviral infections and to compare these studies with clinical observations of infected animals. It is important to remember that these are low dose, time course experiments and our results may differ from other published studies using high infectious doses and examining cells and organs only at the terminal stages of the disease. The highlights of our findings are as follows:

- EBOV infections cause more extensive damage to the blood system than MARV infections.
  - —We observed fibrin thrombi in ZEBOV infections, but not MARV infections, induce the development of DIC.
  - —Rhesus and green monkeys infected with ZEBOV develop clotting; baboons develop hemorrhages; cynomolgus monkeys develop capillary stasis, erythrocyte aggregation, and organs engorged with blood.
- One difference between MARV and EBOV is that EBOV has a non-structural, small, secreted glycoprotein (sGP), which is released from the infected cell. We postulate that the sGP has a role in developing DIC in EBOV-infected animals.
- In our studies, the endothelial cells remained uninfected and structurally unchanged until the animals were near death; therefore, changes in the microcirculation system must be

due to changes induced by the primary target cells, the macrophages. These changes could alter functions for other uninfected cells, including endothelial cells and neutrophils, that may appear structurally unaltered, but we were not able to assess this.

• We postulate that the macrophage mediators, cytokines, are responsible for much of the eventual damage to the microcirculation system, including the microthrombi throughout the visceral organs.

• Blood disorders such as clotting and hemorrhaging are complications in the development of disease and are not the critical pathogenic event. The critical pathogenic event is the disruption of the microcirculation system.

We have further summarized these highlights in the schematic Figure 6-10. In this schematic, we have selected the most evident pathological changes in the blood system, altered microcirculation and damaged hemopoietic systems, and depicted possible mechanisms that may account for these changes. In this scheme, we propose that damage to hemopoietic systems is caused by factors released by macrophages. We have postulated in this scheme that the GP is responsible for DIC in EBOV monkey diseases. We also attribute some of the alterations to the microcirculation system to both macrophage mediator release and to factors released from other cells, specifically endothelial cells and neutrophils.

It is clear that both EBOV and MARV act directly on macrophages. This is substantiated by our electron microscope studies. However, the indirect influences of filoviral infections are major contributors to the lethality of EBOV and MARV diseases. Undoubtedly, the mediators secreted by the infected macrophages have roles in the lethality of filoviruses, but we are unable to study this using only the electron microscope. There is an obvious need for identifying the mediators and then, using electron microscope studies, relating the microcirculation damage they induce with the damage we have seen in our current studies, especially the time course studies. The mechanisms of the macrophage mediator production and release are also critical to understanding how to treat these diseases.

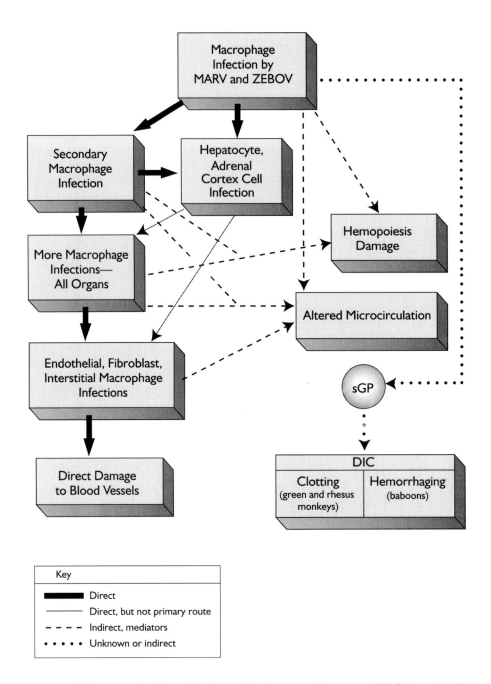

Figure 6-10. Events leading to blood system damage in ZEBOV- and MARV-infected animals. These infections directly and indirectly affect the blood system by infecting macrophages. The endothelial cells of blood vessels are not infected until the last stages of the disease; clotting and hemorrhaging and changes in hemopoiesis result from the cytokines or other substances released by the infected macrophages.

chapter 7

Time Course of the Pathological Changes in Filovirus-Infected Animals

We have discussed how the host is infected by filoviruses, identified the target cells and the organs that are infected, and described how that infection develops over time. In Chapter 5, we examined the changes at the cellular level of the organs over the time course of the infection. In this chapter, we describe the pathological changes to the tissues of these organs over the course of filoviral infection. This is similar to the way we discussed the changes in the blood system in Chapter 6. We studied the time course of the pathological changes in green monkeys infected with relatively small doses of MARV and ZEBOV and in guinea pigs infected with MARV.

We were fortunate to be able to use identical doses of the viruses to enable us to compare the changes caused (1) by two different viruses (MARV and ZEBOV) in the same monkey species, and (2) by MARV in two animal species (guinea pigs and green monkey). In addition, we describe the pathologies we observed for other monkey species infected with ZEBOV. These are the experiments described in Tables 2-1, 4-1 and 6-1. We describe the pathology of each visceral organ (liver, spleen, kidneys, lungs, adrenals, heart, and digestive tract) and the characteristics common to both filoviral diseases in all the studied animals. We also comment on observations that are distinctive among the species. We found that the pathologies are consistent with the microvasculature damage we described in Chapter 6 and can be attributed to factors released in the blood from infected macrophages. Little of the organ damage is attributed to filoviral infections in the parenchyma, except for the liver and adrenal glands, in which case the damage is still secondary to that attributed to the factors in the blood.

Liver

The liver is the main targeted visceral organ in filovirus-infected guinea pigs and monkeys. EBOV and MARV infections have also been shown to alter hepatic functions in humans and other animals; alterations in hepatic functions are reflected in changes in liver enzymes. The hepatic enzymes and bilirubin are elevated in infected humans, and the liver becomes unable to eliminate substances from the body. However, overt jaundice is not common until the terminal stage of the illness [Martini, 1971; Gear, 1975; Peters, 1996; Formenty, 1999]. Similar impairment of hepatic functions was demonstrated in filovirus-infected monkeys. Serum aminotransferases, lactate dehydrogenase, alkaline phosphatase, and creatinine-phosphokinase were elevated in EBOV-infected rhesus monkeys [Fisher-Hoch, 1985; Fisher-Hoch, 1992; Jaax, 1996; Johnson, 1995]. Changes in bilirubin and creatinine contents and changes in the levels of aminotransferases were also reported for ZEBOV-infected baboons [Luchko, 1995; Ryabchikova, 1999a].

Pathological Changes

In the liver, pathological changes for monkeys and guinea pigs involve damage to the blood vessels, filoviral reproduction in hepatocytes and Kuppfer cells, and finally degenerative changes in the hepatocytes. Figure 7-1 shows the liver of a guinea pig infected with MARV before death. The first visible pathological changes in the liver were similar in all animals and resulted from changes in the blood. We observed sinusoid engorgement, stasis, and the formation of rouleaux in blood vessels (Figure 6-1). These changes were visible from days 2 and 3 after the IP inoculation in both

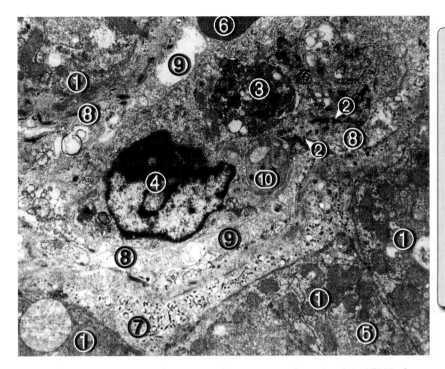

Legend

Figure 7-1

1. Hepatocyte
2. Viral nucleocapsid
3. Phagosome
4. Nucleus
5. Cytoplasm
6. Erythrocyte
7. Disse's space
8. Damaged endothelial cell
9. Sinusoid lumen
10. Thrombocyte

See Note on page xiii.

Figure 7-1. A section of the liver of guinea pig infected with MARV before death (magnification 6,000). The infected Kuppfer cell is located in the sinusoid. The Disse's space contains many viral particles produced by the hepatocytes.

monkeys and guinea pigs and with both ZEBOV and MARV inoculations. Some parts of the liver looked bloodless due to stasis of large blood vessels. We observed swelling of a few endothelial and Kuppfer cells, but as discussed in Chapter 5, this was not directly related to filoviral replication. From day 4 post-inoculation, we observed that the morphologic changes in the liver became prominent and increased in severity up to day 7, at which point the animals usually died. Infected hepatic cells (Kuppfer cells, hepatocytes, and liver endothelial cells) accumulate in the hepatic tissue during the disease. The total number of infected hepatic cells depends both on the infectious dose and on the hepatocyte's structure. As we discussed in Chapter 5, filoviruses were unable to reproduce in abnormal hepatocytes, and we were sometimes unable to find many infected hepatocytes in dystrophic livers. (Summary of figures showing filoviral infections in liver tissue: Figure 4-2 shows a ZEBOV-infected Kuppfer cell; Figure 4-3 shows ZEBOV- and MARV-infected hepatocytes from green monkeys; Figure 5-2 shows a MARV-infected Kuppfer cell; Figure 5-3 shows infected hepatocytes and sinusoids clogged with blood cells; Figure 5-4A shows infected hepatocytes from a ZEBOV-infected baboon; Figure 5-4B shows the liver from a guinea pig infected with MARV; and Figure 5-5 shows the infected liver endothelial cells of a guinea pig infected with MARV.)

Single necrotic macrophages and hepatocytes lie scattered throughout the hepatic parenchyma in the samples obtained from guinea pigs and monkeys on days 4 and 5, post-inoculation. By the terminal stage of the disease, day 7, most sinusoid endothelial and Kuppfer cells were destroyed. Many sinusoids and small vessels were clogged with the erythrocytes and cell debris, as seen in Figure 5-3. In MARV-infected animals, we observed an occasional slight erythrocyte diapedesis occurring into the perisinusoidal Disse's space; normally, only the plasma would be in this space. In ZEBOV-infected green monkeys, the space often contained erythrocytes and fibrin depositions. These are signs of impaired vessel permeability and were usually found in the areas where infected cells were localized. But, the impaired vessels were not themselves infected nor were they necessarily adjacent to infected cells. In ZEBOV-infected green monkeys, fibrin bundles, fibrin thrombi, and mixed fibrin-cellular thrombi were also present in the blood vessels irrespective of virus reproduction in the adjacent cells. Figure 6-6 shows the fibrin clots in the liver from a ZEBOV-infected green monkey; the clots are in the hepatic sinusoids. Figure 7-2 presents another view of fibrin clots; these are in the hepatic sinusoids of a ZEBOV-infected rhesus monkey. ZEBOV infections in green monkeys presented the same as ZEBOV infections in rhesus monkeys.

Many of the uninfected hepatocytes in filovirus-infected animals show swelling of the cytoplasm and mitochondria and show vacuolization of the endoplasmic reticulum. These cells are not associated with the localization of the infected cells, so their dystrophic changes may be related to toxic influences. Large areas of dead hepatocytes are not seen, but small accumulations of destroyed hepatocytes are present in the liver at the terminal stages. In general, the formation of large necrotic foci, involving

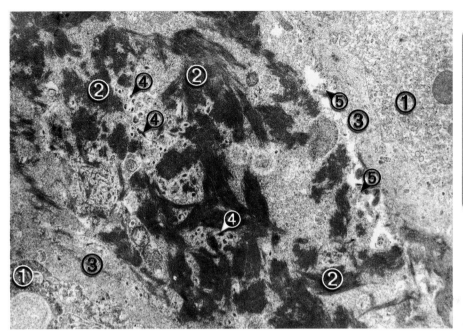

Legend

Figure 7-2
1. Hepatocyte
2. Fibrin
3. Disse's space
4. Viral particle
5. Destroyed
   sinusoid lining

See Note on page xiii.

Figure 7-2. Fibrin thrombus clogging a hepatic sinusoid in a rhesus monkey infected with ZEBOV (magnification 10,500). The liver has a very extensive blood flow and the fibrin thrombi that clog the sinusoids alter that blood flow. The thrombi make a mesh that hinders the blood cleaning function of the liver.

several lobules of the liver, was not typical of the liver damage observed in animals infected with MARV and ZEBOV.

Our time course comparison of liver samples shows the cumulative pathological changes of the hepatic parenchyma and vascular system in filovirus-infected guinea pigs and monkeys. The cumulative damage is consistent with the biochemical data for liver damage. However, although the liver is affected in filoviral infections, the level of hepatic damage is incomparably smaller than that seen in fulminant viral hepatitis; therefore, hepatic damage cannot be the direct cause of death in filovirus-infected humans and animals.

The pathological changes we observed in ZEBOV-infected monkey livers, baboons, rhesus, and cynomolgus monkeys, generally depend on the pattern of the vasculature impairment. Baboon livers show hemorrhages (as shown in Figure 7-3), while those of rhesus and green monkeys show fibrin clots (as shown in Figure 7-2). Cynomolgus monkey livers appear the least damaged (i.e., prominent fibrin depositions and hemorrhages are absent), but these livers have the highest number of ZEBOV-infected cells. Of course, if the animals are inoculated with large infectious doses of EBOV (10^5 LD_{50}), there is massive liver damage in all monkey species and such details would not be noticed [Murphy, 1971; Baskerville, 1978; Baskerville, 1985; Jaax, 1996; Johnson, 1995].

Legend

Figure 7-3

1. Hepatocyte

2. Endothelial cell

3. Intravascular erythrocyte

4. Erythrocyte outside blood vessel

5. Sinusoid lining

6. Lumen

7. Viral inclusion

See Note on page xiii.

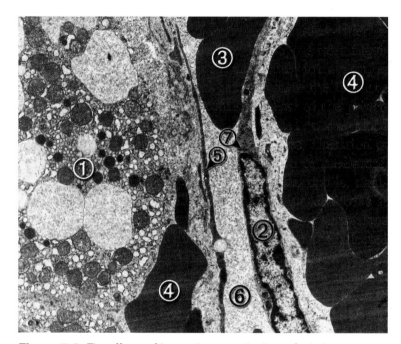

Figure 7-3. The effects of hemorrhages in the liver of a baboon infected with ZEBOV (magnification 7,000). The erythrocytes have accumulated outside the sinusoids.

Inflammation

Inflammation is normally an important part of any infectious disease's pathological process and is essential in initiating immune defenses. Typically, it is characterized by the presence of leukocytes and their accumulation in the infected tissues. However, the absence of inflammatory reaction in the infected organs is characteristic of the filoviral diseases. All of the researchers who examined the organs of filovirus-infected animals and humans have noted the lack of leukocyte infiltration in the infected liver. In many other viral infections associated with hepatic changes and damage, leukocytes accumulate in the liver during the first 5 days and the number of natural killer cells in hepatic tissue increases 5–50 fold. In the next step, virus-specific T-lymphocytes aggregate in the liver and clear the virus from the organ [McIntyre, 1986; McIntyre, 1988; Mena, 2000; Pilaro, 1994]. The lack of leukocyte infiltration strongly suggests that the immune system's defense fails during filoviral disease.

The liver of filovirus-infected animals is the best organ in which to look for an inflammatory reaction because it contains the largest number of infected cells and viral particles. In our studies, we observed no inflammatory reaction in the liver of MARV and ZEBOV-infected green monkeys. There were neither neutrophils nor mononuclear cells near the infected hepatocytes. The same effect was observed in ZEBOV-infected baboons, rhesus, and cynomolgus monkeys. We were fortunate to be able to compare the lack of inflammation in livers from ZEBOV-infected monkeys with those from guinea pigs. Our previous work has established that non-lethal Ebola disease occurs in guinea pigs, but after sequential passages of the virus in guinea pigs, ZEBOV adapted to the guinea pigs and became fatal. The unadapted ZEBOV induces pronounced focal inflammation in the liver. This can be seen in Figure 7-4, where the accumulation of leukocytes indicates the immune system is working to eliminate the infected cells. The photographs (Figures 5-3 and 6-1) of ZEBOV-infected monkey livers show the absence of inflammation [Pereboeva, 1993; Ryabchikova, 1993; Ryabchikova, 1996].

We compared the two routes of MARV infection in guinea pigs, IP inoculation vs. aerosolized inoculation. With an infectious dose of 2–5 LD_{50} using aerosolized MARV, viremia occurred in 72 hours

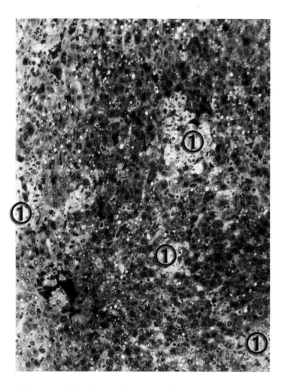

Figure 7-4. Image from a light microscope showing the liver from a guinea pig infected with unadapted ZEBOV. The inflammatory foci are visible. The foci are an accumulation of leukocytes, which are fighting the infected cells. Normally, local inflammations are a defensive reaction of the immune system and will eventually eliminate the infected cells.

(see Table 4-1 for dose, mode, and time to viremia). In guinea pigs infected with MARV (IP inoculation), the neutrophils (the major leukocytes in the inflammatory response) occasionally accumulated in sinusoids near the infected cells; however, we did not observe neutrophils that migrated from the bloodstream nor did we observe neutrophils that attacked the infected cells. In guinea pigs infected by the aerosol route, we were able to detect the migration of leukocytes from blood vessels and their contact with infected hepatocytes. These features are shown in Figure 7-5, where the leukocytes attack the MARV-infected hepatocytes. However, we did not observe any signs that the infected cells were killed [Ryabchikova, 1996a]. Based on these data, we suggest that

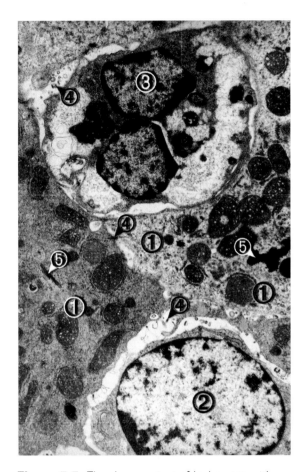

Legend

Figure 7-5
1. Hepatocyte
2. Lymphocyte
3. Neutrophil
4. Viral particle
5. Viral inclusion

See Note on page xiii.

Figure 7-5. The close contact of leukocytes with infected hepatocytes from the liver of a guinea pig infected by aerosolized MARV (magnification 6,200). The leukocytes appear to actually attack the infected hepatocyte. The attack is ineffective because MARV is fatal to guinea pigs.

there may be some factor(s) preventing neutrophil accumulation and defense operations in the infected liver. When these factors are delayed (e.g., the delay that occurs from an aerosol infection), the leukocytes begin to operate, but when the factors appear in the blood, the operation stops and neutrophil defense ceases. The factors may be host or viral in nature and seem to be related to the delay of MARV entry into the bloodstream.

Our morphologic studies of the livers of filovirus-infected animals revealed marked damage of the hepatic structure. The primary causes were changes in the blood supply, filoviral reproduction, and toxic influences. These factors, combined with variations in the hepatic structure, determine the individual differences between animals infected with ZEBOV and MARV. The difference in hepatic pathomorphology between monkey species infected with ZEBOV is determined by the pattern of organ vasculature damage (e.g., hemorrhages in the baboon liver and fibrin deposition in rhesus and green monkey livers). Hepatic lesions have a diffuse character and, in monkeys or guinea pigs fatally infected with ZEBOV and MARV, there are no signs of inflammatory reactions.

Spleen

Although the liver is the target organ, the spleen (due to the higher concentration of macrophages) is the organ most affected in MARV- and EBOV-infected animals, regardless of the infectious dose, animal species, and mode of virus inoculation. The two major components of the spleen are the red pulp involved in filtering the blood and the white pulp involved in immunological functions. Most of the blood in an organism passes through the spleen, and the spleen acts as a reservoir for the blood as it brings the blood into contact with lymphocytes and removes used and damaged blood components. Consequently, damage or changes to the blood and factors released in the blood are likely to have the greatest effect on the spleen compared to other organs. We expect to see high concentrations of neutrophils and macrophages in the red pulp because these are the cells that will remove waste by phagocytosis. In this section, we discuss the time course changes in the spleen's red pulp; the spleen's white pulp is involved in immunity and time course changes in the white pulp will be described in Chapter 8, "Immunopathology."

We observed that pathological changes in splenic red pulp appeared during the first 3 days in ZEBOV- and MARV-infected animals. Sections of the red pulp displayed evidence of hemostasis, pronounced engorgement of venules and sinuses, and thrombosis. Figure 7-6 contains an example of the type of

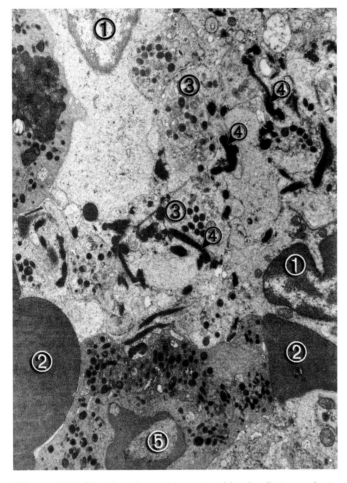

Legend

Figure 7-6

1. Lymphocyte
2. Erythrocyte
3. Thrombocyte
4. Fibrin clump
5. Neutrophil

See Note on page xiii.

Figure 7-6. The thrombus with various blood cells in a splenic red pulp vessel (magnification 8,000). This pathology is typical for clotting.

thrombus we observed in the spleen. Typically, the thrombus contained fibrin clumps and thrombocytes or platelets. From the early stages of the infection, we noted the accumulation of tremendous numbers of neutrophils in the red pulp. The splenic parenchyma appeared to be literally soaked with the neutrophils and erythrocytes. Some neutrophils contained lucid zones in the cytoplasm, corresponding to the sites where lysosome enzymes were liberated.

An avalanche of pathological changes developed in the red pulp in monkeys and guinea pigs from days 4 to 5 post-inoculation. Infected macrophage cells, mostly related to splenic sinuses, were scattered throughout the tissue, as seen in Figure 7-7 from a ZEBOV-infected green monkey. The macrophages and cells lining the sinuses became swollen, and many disintegrated. This made it difficult to distinguish the blurred borders of the sinuses and vessels. The lumens of spleen's sinuses and small blood vessels were clogged with blood cells. Disorders in blood vessel permeability were evidenced not only by diapedesis of the erythrocytes through vessel walls, but also by fibrin depositions surrounding the blood vessels (Figure 6-8). In ZEBOV-infected green monkeys, fibrin thrombi, fibrin masses, and bundles were deposited in sinus and vascular lumina and outside the vessels. Some of these features can be seen in Figure 7-8. In particular, thrombocytes

Legend

Figure 7-7

1. Nucleus

2. Mitochondria

3. Viral inclusion body with dense nucleocapsids

4. Phagosome

See Note on page xiii.

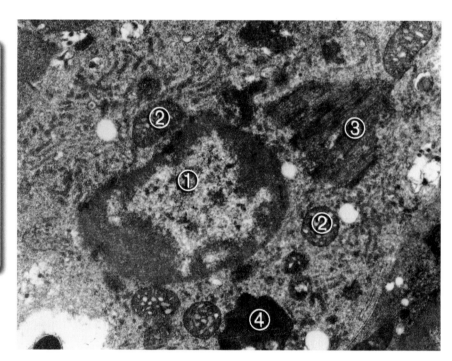

Figure 7-7. A ZEBOV-infected macrophage in the splenic red pulp of a green monkey (magnification 16,000). This is typical of the images we observed in the spleen. The phagosomes and viral inclusions can be seen in the infected macrophage.

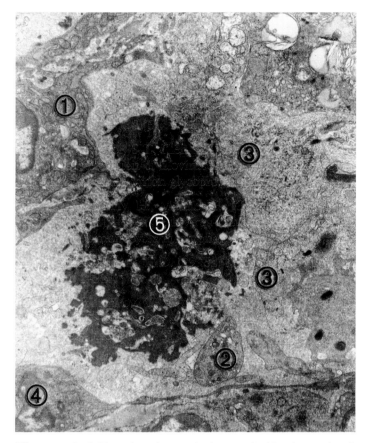

Legend

Figure 7-8
1. Macrophage
2. Thrombocyte
3. Defective thrombocyte
4. Endothelial cell
5. Fibrin

See Note on page xiii.

Figure 7-8. A fibrin thrombus in the lumen of a blood vessel in the red pulp of a ZEBOV-infected green monkey (magnification 6,000). Damage to the spleen eventually results in the loss of its characteristic architecture. At the microscopic scale, the tissue becomes a mass of cell debris, fibrin, neutrophils, and erythrocytes.

without apparent granules were common. The red pulp splenic tissue in ZEBOV-infected green monkeys was sometimes devoid of cells, in which case it had the appearance of large cavities filled with fibrin clumps and bundles, and masses and stray erythrocytes. In the spleens of MARV-infected animals, fibrin also clumped outside the vessels, but in smaller amounts. At the disease's terminal stages, the splenic red pulp generally lost its distinctive architecture to such a degree that it became unrecognizable. The tissue became a continuous conglomerate of cell debris, fibrin, erythrocytes, and neutrophils. Figure 7-9 shows part of a green monkey's splenic red pulp during the terminal stages of ZEBOV infection, where the sinuses have widened to accommodate the erythrocytes, fibrin, and cell debris. Some of the cell debris contains groups of virus particles indicating that the cell debris is likely to be from an infected macrophage. Blood could barely, if at all, pass through the tissue because of all the debris

Legend

Figure 7-9

1. Sinus endothelial lining
2. Fibrin
3. Neutrophil
4. Erythrocyte
5. Cellular debris
6. Lymphocyte

See Note on page xiii.

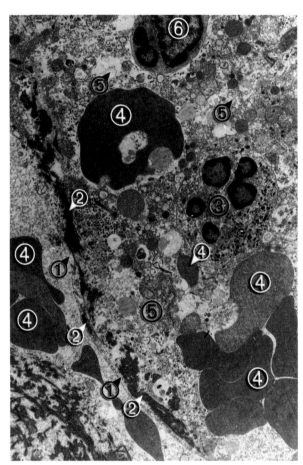

Figure 7-9. Part of a green monkey's splenic red pulp illustrating the main features of spleen damage in the terminal stages of ZEBOV infection (magnification 3,500). The left corner shows widened sinus containing erythrocytes and fibrin. Endothelial lining of the sinus can be seen. Fibrin deposits make a contour from the outer side of the sinus. The other portion of the picture is filled by cellular debris and contains erythrocytes, neutrophils, and lymphocytes. This debris may be from a destroyed macrophage because of the accumulation of ZEBOV particles.

and fibrin. This description represents the most pronounced stage of splenic lesions, and it is typical for green monkeys infected with ZEBOV in a dose of 100 LD_{50}. Green monkeys infected with MARV in the same dose displayed a lesser degree of lesions. The pathology of the splenic red pulp in guinea pigs infected with 100 LD_{50} of MARV was advanced, similar to the damage shown in Figure 7-9. Rhesus monkeys infected with ZEBOV developed damage identical to that in green monkeys infected with the same doses of ZEBOV. Splenic red pulp in baboons showed severe damage comparable with that in green and rhesus monkeys but differed by having a more pronounced hemorrhagic component.

In contrast to the liver, the number of the infected cells in splenic red pulp decreased during filoviral infection. Of the cells in the spleen, we observed that only the macrophages are able to support filoviral reproduction. Once these infected cells are destroyed, new macrophages are not formed and newly infected cells do not appear. The pathological changes in splenic red pulp of ZEBOV and MARV-infected animals correspond to the most outstanding consequences of the damage in the blood system.

Kidneys

The kidneys are one of the other major organs that have extended contact with blood, and consequently, we expect considerable damage to the kidneys during filoviral diseases. This is consistent with the changes in kidney functions observed during filoviral disease of both humans and monkeys. The pattern of renal changes and damage in filovirus-infected monkeys is similar to that found in infected humans. The plasma levels of urea and creatinine and the activities of lactate dehydrogenases and creatinine phosphokinase all have been reported to increase, while sodium, potassium, and calcium levels decrease in rhesus monkeys during Ebola disease [Fisher-Hoch, 1985; Jaax, 1996; Johnson, 1995]. A considerable increase in the urea and creatinine content was found in ZEBOV-infected baboons [Luchko, 1995; Ryabchikova, 1999a]. However, the acute renal insufficiency was not recorded, and despite the damage from filoviral infections, injury of the kidney is not suspected as a direct cause of death.

The pathological changes in the kidneys of filovirus-infected monkeys are extensive when large infectious doses are administered. The morphological pattern of kidney impairment consists of damage to the blood vessels and kidney cells. The earliest changes appeared on day 3 post-inoculation. These changes were focal stasis and thrombosis of capillaries between the tubules and, in the glomerule, edema of some endothelial cells. Figure 6-1B shows the erythrocyte thrombi in the blood vessels of the kidney. Podocytes, the epithelial cells in the glomerular capillaries of the kidney, remained morphologically unchanged, while many cells of the proximal tubules showed dystrophic changes. These cells had disorganized basal folds and apical microvilli. Dystrophic changes in the epithelial cells, swelling of the cytoplasm and mitochondria, developed in the distal tubules 2 to 3 days later.

Pronounced pathological changes involving large areas of the parenchyma were observed in the kidneys from day 5 post-inoculation. The sections showed the capillaries were clogged with erythrocytes; endothelial cells had degenerated and only the basal membrane was present in some sites. In ZEBOV-infected green monkeys, fibrin deposits were found in capillaries, small vessels, and in the pericapillary spaces. The focal pattern of kidney damage is clearly visible in the light microscope. Figure 7-10A shows both necrotic and unaltered glomeruli in the same section. At the electron microscopic level, other changes were observed. Although uninfected, various patterns of dystrophic and necrotic changes can be seen in the podocytes in Figure 7-10B. In Figure 7-11A, the lumens of the tubules are seen to contain cell debris and few erythrocytes. In Figure 7-11B, mineral salts can also be seen. Most of the tubular epithelial cells in the affected kidney zones were altered, but uninfected. We observed necrotic areas in the kidney tissues; some of these areas were light (absence of material), whereas some areas were dark (accumulation of stained material). We observed swelling of the cytoplasm and organelles in the light area and marked condensation in the dark areas. Although there was damage to all the blood vessels in the kidney, the specific type of damage was species dependent; the prevalence of hemorrhages and fibrin deposits in ZEBOV-infected monkeys followed the same pattern as the blood damage in the other organs.

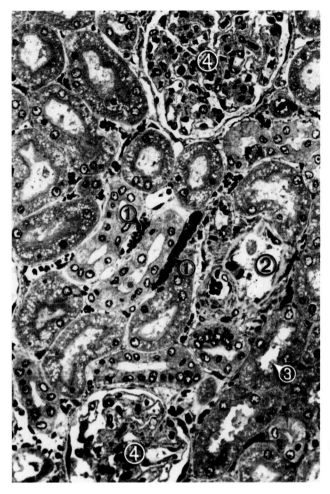

Legend

Figure 7-10

1. Erythrocyte
2. Necrosis
3. Proximal tubule
4. Glomerulus
5. Basal membrane
6. Glomerulus space
7. Destroyed endothelium
8. Neutrophil
9. Podocyte
10. Degenerating podocyte

See Note on page xiii.

Figure 7-10A

Figure 7-10. Renal damage in green monkeys infected with MARV via a semithin light microscope section and an ultrathin electron microscope section. **Figure 7-10A** shows a semithin section of the kidney of a green monkey infected with MARV seen with a light microscope. **Figure 7-10B** (page 148) shows part of the glomerulus under the electron microscope (magnification 15,000). Renal damage in filovirus-infected animals is not caused by the viral replication in the kidney epithelial cells. Changes in the blood circulation and accumulation of toxic metabolites are the main cause of the damage. The changes in blood circulation accentuate the changes from the endothelial cell damage and the final result is pronounced lesions in the kidney tissue and altered renal functions.

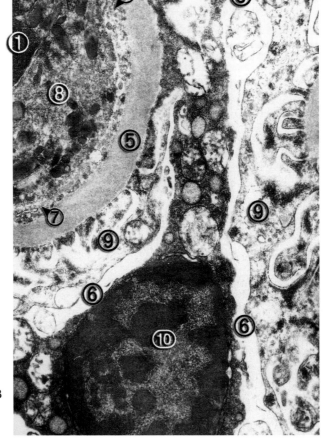

Figure 7-10B

Figure 7-10. . . . Figure 7-10B shows part of the glomerulus under the electron microscope (magnification 15,000). Renal damage in filovirus-infected animals is not caused by the viral replication in the kidney epithelial cells. Changes in the blood circulation and accumulation of toxic metabolites are the main cause of the damage. The changes in blood circulation accentuate the changes from the endothelial cell damage and the final result is pronounced lesions in the kidney tissue and altered renal functions.

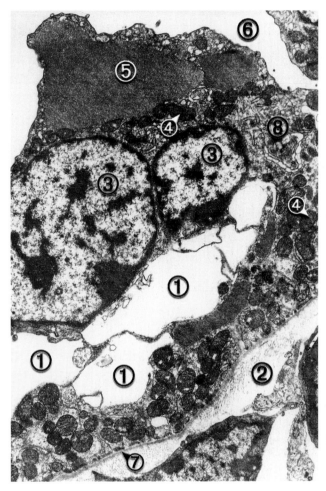

Legend

Figure 7-11

1. Vacuole
2. Interstitial tissue
3. Nucleus
4. Mitochondria
5. Inclusion of protein material
6. Lumen of tubule
7. Basal membrane
8. Cytoplasm
9. Mineral salt
10. Endothelial cell

See Note on page xiii.

Figure 7-11A

Figure 7-11. Two variations of the type of localized renal tissue lesions that are seen in filovirus-infected animals. **Figure 7-11A** shows the damage to the renal tubules (magnification 7,700). **Figure 7-11B** (page 150) shows a mineral salt deposit in the proximal tubule of the kidney (8,000).

Legend

Figure 7-11

1. Vacuole

2. Interstitial tissue

3. Nucleus

4. Mitochondria

5. Inclusion of
   protein material

6. Lumen of tubule

7. Basal
   membrane

8. Cytoplasm

9. Mineral salt

10. Endothelial cell

See Note on page xiii.

Figure 7-11B

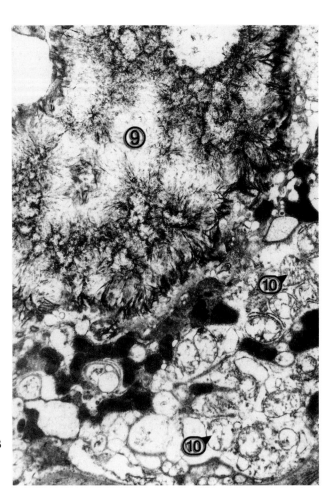

Figure 7-11. . . . **Figure 7-11B** shows a mineral salt deposit in the proximal tubule of the kidney (8,000).

Thus, our kidney studies revealed pronounced damage to the renal tubular system and glomeruli in monkeys infected with MARV or ZEBOV. In guinea pigs infected with MARV, the pattern of the pathological changes in kidneys was the same as in monkeys, but far less marked. Our morphological studies show that kidney damage is not related directly to filoviral reproduction within the kidneys themselves. The pattern is that of cytotoxic damage and hematologic disorders. Both factors are closely related and accentuate each other during the disease.

Lungs

We examined lung tissue for the pathologies that developed over the course of the disease. Our time course studies did not reveal morphological evidence of pneumonia or bronchitis caused by the filoviruses in the monkeys and guinea pigs.* On days 4 to 5 post-inoculation, the lungs became congested with blood, and we saw mild perivascular edema and small aggregates of neutrophils and platelets in blood vessels. Such microvasculature damage occurred both in the upper and lower respiratory tracts. Diapedesis of the erythrocytes and pronounced accumulation of the neutrophils in alveolar capillaries and small vessels developed later in the course of disease. This was shown in Figures 6-3 and 6-8. This pattern of pathological changes remained unchanged up until the deaths of the monkeys and guinea pigs infected with MARV.

In ZEBOV-infected green monkeys, this pattern was exaggerated by fibrin deposits in the blood vessels and interstitial space.

Special note: Some lung impairment in filovirus-infected animals may be associated with non-specific damage to lungs, especially in monkeys. During our examinations of lung tissue pathologies, we found evidence in wild monkeys and sometimes in guinea pigs of various acute and chronic respiratory diseases separate from lesions and morphologies attributed to filoviruses. The presence of these nonspecific lung alterations makes it difficult to examine the changes from filoviral injury, especially when high infectious doses are used. The pneumonia reported in some EBOV-infected monkeys may have been caused by the virus or by other agents [Johnson, 1995]. Concurrent infections may explain the variability in the pattern of lung damage in filovirus-infected monkeys described in other reports [Baskerville, 1978; Baskerville 1985; Murphy, 1971].

Edema and necrosis of many endothelial cells, alveolar cells, and alveolar basal membrane occurred, as is shown in Figure 7-12 (see Figure 5-7 for comparison of the sizes of the basal membrane). In some rare cases, infected alveolar and bronchial epithelial cells were found at the terminal stages in filoviral diseases. The pattern of lung pathological changes we observed demonstrates a lack of inflammation and is further evidence for severe disorders in microcirculation. Microcirculation was impaired throughout the entire pulmonary tissue in filovirus-infected animals and this obviously altered the gas-exchange functions in the lungs and subsequently the blood oxygen supply.

Legend

Figure 7-12

1. Basal membrane
2. Alveolar space
3. Alveolar cell
4. Interstitial tissue
5. Erythrocyte

See Note on page xiii.

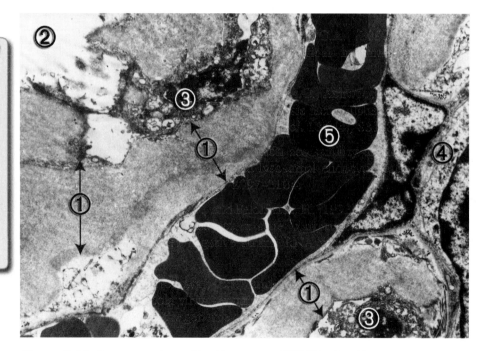

Figure 7-12. Damage to the air-blood barrier in a ZEBOV-infected green monkey (magnification 4,000). This is an important picture showing the severe damage of the lung tissue, which alters the gas exchange to the organism. Such damage is undoubtedly life threatening. The basal membrane providing transport of oxygen to blood is widened to a large extent due to edema. (For comparison, Figure 5-7 shows an infected macrophage in an alveolar capillary where the basal membrane is more normal in size.) (Photo by Dr. L. Kolesnikova)

We did not observe ZEBOV and MARV replication in lung respiratory epithelium except in rare cases. Thus, the infection of the respiratory epithelium is not the cause for most of the damage affecting the respiratory lining responsible for air-blood exchange. The primary factor influencing lung functions appears to be the damage to the microvasculature system in the capillaries and venules of the lung.

Adrenals

We examined the effect of filoviral infections on the adrenal glands. We were able to conduct a time course study of changes in the pathology of adrenal glands in monkeys infected with ZEBOV, but not with MARV. In MARV-infected monkeys and guinea pigs, we examined the adrenals only at the terminal stages. The picture we observed in MARV infections corresponded to those in ZEBOV-infected green monkeys, but as with other organs, MARV infections produced a smaller level of damage.

Green monkeys infected with ZEBOV showed early damage to adrenals; by days 2 to 3 post-inoculation, we noted some capillaries of the cortex were congested with blood and we occasionally saw platelets adhering to the vascular wall. A decrease in the number of lipid droplets was observed in the zona fasciculata cells on day 3 post-inoculation. Lesions accumulated during the disease, and on day 4 post-inoculation, we could observe small foci of erythrocyte diapedesis and extracapillary deposition of fibrin fibers in the adrenal cortex. From day 5, we observed necrosis of few cells and phagocytosis of cellular debris by neutrophils. Fibrin thrombi were found in the blood vessels as seen in Figure 6-2B. In most zona fasciculata cells, there was a decrease in the number of lipid droplets and we observed the appearance of large mitochondria with lysed cristae (inward folds) and matrices. Occasional degranulation of parenchymal cells was seen in the adrenal medulla. Thus, monkey adrenals do not exhibit prominent necrotic changes, but the morphology of the organ is evidence for marked impairment in the hormone-producing function.

As we described in Chapter 4, the adrenals are the second organ, after the liver, whose parenchyma supports replication of MARV and ZEBOV. Filoviruses replicate in the adrenal cortical cells of green monkeys. We also observed filoviral replication in fibroblasts and endothelial cells in the adrenals of the infected monkeys. In Figure 4-4, we can see the viral particles in green monkey adrenal cortical cells. Figure 7-13 shows the viral inclusions and viral particles in the adrenal cortex cells and in adrenal fibroblasts of ZEBOV-infected green monkeys. These same target

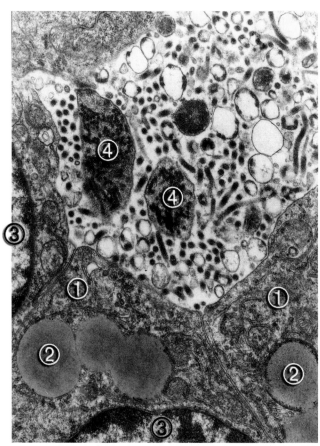

Legend

Figure 7-13

1. Cytoplasm

2. Lipid droplet

3. Nucleus of adrenal cortex cell

4. Viral inclusion

5. Viral particle

6. Fibroblast

7. Basal membrane

8. Adrenal cortex cell

9. Fibroblast protrusion with viral particle

See Note on page xiii.

Figure 7-13A

Figure 7-13. ZEBOV reproduction in the adrenal glands of a green monkey. **Figure 7-13A** shows the cortical cells and a section of adjacent cells producing many viral particles located in the intercellular space (magnification 32,000). Sections of the cellular protrusions filled with viral nucleocapsids can be seen. **Figure 7-13B** shows an adrenal fibroblast of interstitial tissue infected with ZEBOV (magnification 16,800). Fibroblast protrusions containing viral nucleocapsids can be seen.

cells were observed in all studied monkey species infected with ZEBOV. As with the liver, the infected adrenals demonstrated all of the species-specific differences we observed in damage to the blood system. Green and rhesus monkeys showed fibrin deposits associated with clotting as seen in Figure 6-2A, while baboon adrenals developed prominent hemorrhages.

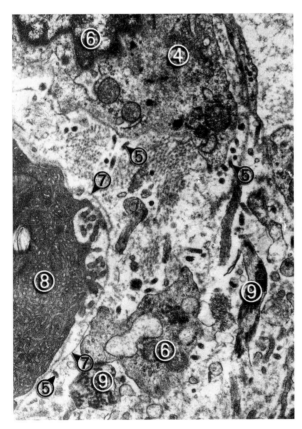

Figure 7-13B

Descriptions of the adrenal damage in filovirus-infected animals are meager in published articles. Hemorrhages and diffuse necrosis in the fascicular zone at the terminal stage in rhesus and cynomolgus monkeys infected with ZEBOV and REBOV, respectively, have been reported [Baskerville, 1978; Geisbert, 1992; Jaax, 1996]. Although damage to the adrenals has been documented in filoviral diseases, there have been no studies on the effects of the filoviral infection on hormone-producing functions, either in animals or humans. Our electron microscopic examination revealed a significant decrease in the number of lipid droplets in the adrenal cortical cells, which is indicative of depressed hormone-producing functions. This depression may be very significant in the pathogenesis of filoviral diseases because hormones produced by the adrenal cortex include those with anti-inflammatory properties. Moreover, adrenal hormones, such as cortisol, which are released in response to hemorrhage, help to mediate fluid exchange and restore blood volume. Disruption of adrenal functions may have significant effects in the pathogenesis of filoviral disease.

Heart

Although the macrophage and blood are primary targets in filoviral infections, we examined the heart muscle only in ZEBOV-infected monkeys. ZEBOV infections produce greater damage than MARV infections; therefore, if the damage was not extensive and significant in ZEBOV infections, there would be little additional knowledge gained by examining the tissues in MARV infections. We observed congestion of blood vessels, small foci of diapedesis of the erythrocytes, intravascular and perivascular deposition of fibrin, and swelling of few endothelial cells from day 3 post-inoculation. These changes increased over the course of disease. Necrosis of infected endothelial cells was found at the terminal stages. Small foci of lysed myofibrils, cristae, and mitochondrial matrix, presumably due to disturbed microcirculation, developed in cardiomyocytes. Figure 7-14 shows some of the changes in heart tissue. Despite the damage to the blood system, heart muscle itself was not significantly damaged. These data clearly

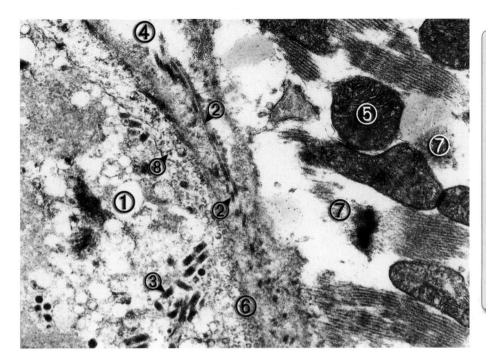

Legend

Figure 7-14
1. Lumen
2. Collagen fiber
3. Viral particle
4. Interstitial tissue
5. Muscle cell
6. Destroyed endothelial cell
7. Lysed myofibril
8. Endothelial cell

See Note on page xiii.

Figure 7-14. A section from the heart of green monkey infected with ZEBOV (magnification 21,000). The neighboring blood vessel (left part) and cardiac muscle cell (right part) are separated with interstitial tissue. Vessel lumen contains cellular debris and viral particles. The muscle cell shows normal mitochondria and lysed myofibrils. (Photo by Dr. L. Kolesnikova)

show that the pattern of pathological changes in the heart is mainly due to microcirculatory disturbances.

Digestive Tract

Microscopic examination of the stomach and intestines, pancreas, and salivary glands in MARV and ZEBOV-infected monkeys and guinea pigs did not reveal any marked changes in the architecture of the mucous layer and gland structure. Pathological changes were observed in the lamina propria, but these were changes and damage to the blood capillaries and small vessels. Only minor changes were found in guinea pigs; their vessels showed rouleaux in the lumens and rare erythrocyte thrombi in the small venules. There were signs of impaired hemostasis in monkey intestines, common for all organs, and most conspicuous in Ebola diseases. Small hemorrhages, fibrin thrombi and single fibrin bundles in blood vessels, and edema of few endothelial cells were sometimes observed in monkey lamina propria at the terminal stages of filoviral disease. Damage became more pronounced as the infectious dose increased; however, apparent pathological changes in the epithelium did not develop. Our observations of the intestine are in agreement with other reported data on pathological changes in rhesus monkeys infected with EBOV [Baskerville, 1978; Baskerville, 1985; Jaax, 1996] and cynomolgus monkeys infected with REBOV [Geisbert, 1992].

Summary

Our time course studies of the visceral organs of guinea pigs and green monkeys infected with MARV and ZEBOV revealed common features in the pattern of pathological changes. From the early days of infection, microcirculatory disturbances were the primary changes in all the organs of all the animals. Microcirculation damage appears to be the most significant cause for the development of dystrophic changes in the visceral organs. The most severe damage was noted in liver, spleen, kidneys, lungs, and adrenals of all the infected animals. The lack of inflammation in the visceral organs is another common feature of filoviral diseases and is a clue as to the role of the immune system in the progress of filoviral infections. The pathological changes in MARV infections are similar for both monkeys and guinea pigs, but the degree of damage in monkeys was greater than in guinea pigs. The degree of damage in general was greater in ZEBOV infections than in MARV infections.

chapter 8

Immunopathology

It is natural to first notice the most outstanding and impressive features of any phenomenon. The most impressive features of filoviral diseases are blood damage, prostration, fever, and very rapid death. With these compelling signs, scientists did not at first notice other aspects of the disease, especially something as subtle as changes in the immune system. Researchers noted that the host died but generally did not focus on the immune response in fatal filoviral infections [Peters, 1996; Siegert, 1972].

Although filoviruses replicate in macrophages, hepatocytes, and adrenal cortical cells, we did not find pathological evidence to indicate that viruses simply kill these infected cells. To the contrary, most of the damage caused by the viruses appears to be indirect. Many viruses cause disease and damage by indirect effects (e.g., poliovirus, paramyxovirus, and herpes viruses). These indirect effects are called immunopathology and refer to the damage done to and by the immune system.

We began our studies of filoviral infections more than a decade ago, before the more modern methods for examining immunity using commercial kits had been widely introduced into research practice. In fact, even today there is no comprehensive, general method to evaluate the state of immunity in an organism as a whole. Of course we cannot examine the different cytokines and other factors released during the immunological response with the electron microscope. But using microscopy, it is possible to compare the same morphological parameters characteristic of immunological reactions in different animals and different organs. Perhaps these parameters seem too coarse for examining a system controlled by molecules, but morphological parameters are reliable for a general study of the immunity impairment and for outlining a direction for subsequent investigations.

We used microscopy to examine samples of lymphatic tissue obtained during our time course filoviral studies and combined these results with information from our other studies. The data presented in this chapter were obtained using more than 100 animals and represent only those parameters characteristic of immune system damage common to all MARV- and ZEBOV-infected animals. Unique or rare findings are not presented.

As we saw in the previous chapters, the filoviruses cause damage far beyond the macrophages they first infect. The infected macrophages are transported to the rest of the organs via the blood and lymph circulatory systems. Those organs in which the blood and lymph have the greatest contact with (spleen and lymph nodes) are those in which we would expect to see the most damage. Lymphocytes are formed in the bone marrow and the immature lymphocytes can be found in the lymph nodes. When activated by an infection, the immature lymphocytes differentiate to form a specific or lymphocyte-mediated response. We found that in the filoviral infections, there was no evidence that this differentiation occurred. It is well known that the inflammatory response is an important and even infection-controlling part of the immune response to viral infections. As we have noted throughout our discussions, we found evidence that the inflammatory response was impaired; we often found no accumulation of large lymphocytes and neutrophils in damaged tissues. We looked at the morphological aspects of the lymphatic system to understand the changes that occurred to the immune system.

Filoviral Reproduction In Lymphatic Tissue

We examined the lymphoid tissue from all anatomical locations: splenic white pulp; mesenteric, inguinal, and peribronchial lymph nodes; lymphoid nodules; and follicles of the respiratory and the gastrointestinal tracts. We collected samples daily from green monkeys and guinea pigs fatally infected with MARV and ZEBOV.

The first MARV-infected macrophages of lymphatic tissue appeared in the blood vessels of the splenic white pulp and mesenteric lymph nodes on day 4 post-inoculation in both guinea pigs and green monkeys. The first ZEBOV-infected macrophages were detected in the splenic white pulp on day 3 and in the lymph nodes on day 4 post-inoculation. These infected macrophages showed all the characteristic morphological signs for filoviral infection: viral inclusions, nucleocapsids, and viral particles near the cell. These can be seen in Figure 8-1, a photograph of a ZEBOV-infected macrophage from the lymph node of a green monkey. The net-like structures often seen in ZEBOV infection are also visible. The number of infected macrophages in the lymphatic tissue was relatively small, even at the terminal stages. Occasionally, we found no infected macrophages in the lymphatic follicles of the intestines or respiratory tract. Not all macrophages were infected by filoviruses, even in animals infected with high doses. For example, we did not observe reproduction of MARV and ZEBOV in macrophages in the medullar zones of lymph nodes. Presumably this discrimination of macrophages by filoviruses is related to the heterogeneity of the macrophage population.

Frequently, the fibroblasts and endothelial cells of lymphatic tissue were not infected with the filoviruses, but there were often infected fibroblasts in the connective tissue surrounding the lymph nodes and in the lymphatic follicles. We never saw lymphocytes infected with ZEBOV and MARV.

Pathological Changes

We found morphologic changes in the lymphatic tissue very early in the infections in all animals. The animals stopped forming new lymphocytes and stopped their differentiation into mature lymphocytes with specific immune responses; this means that the cell-mediated immune response was not developed. Within a few days, the lymphocytes were depleted, even though the lymphocytes do not support filoviral infection. We also noted that macrophages and stromal cells were altered but not necessarily

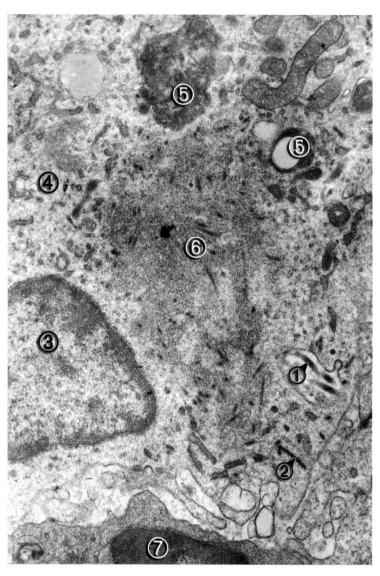

Figure 8-1

1. Viral particle
2. Nucleocapsid
3. Nucleus
4. Cytoplasm
5. Phagosome
6. Viral inclusion
7. Lymphocyte

See Note on page xiii.

Figure 8-1. A ZEBOV-infected macrophage in the lymphatic node of green monkey with all the hallmarks of a filoviral infection (magnification 16,000).

destroyed. The dendritic cells were small in number and so difficult to count and observe in a representative fashion, but we noted that by the terminal stages of the disease, most of these were destroyed. The lack of lymphocyte differentiation and cell-mediated immune response development indicates that the immune system was altered by the filoviral infections.

Formation of Lymphocytes

Within 2 or 3 days post-inoculation, we no longer could find mitosis in lymphatic cells or any visible signs of differentiation of the lymphocytes and formation of plasma cells in any of the lymphatic tissue in green monkeys and guinea pigs. These observations indicate that the development of specific immune responses to filoviral infection was blocked or at least not activated. These morphological signs of the lack of a specific immune response persisted during the course of the disease and regardless of whether or not filovirus-infected cells were detected in the lymphatic organ sections.

What causes this lack of initiation of specific immune response? We hypothesize that a humoral agent or agents released at the early stages of the infection, probably by infected macrophages, in some manner blocks the activation of the specific immune response.

What about mitosis in other types of cells? Are these also blocked or inhibited? We examined the intestinal epithelium in filovirus-infected animals, and we observed normal mitosis. So, it appears that whatever factors are involved, the inactivation or blockage of mitosis in lymphocytes is selective and intended specifically for lymphoid cells.

Lymphoid Depletion

Lymphoid depletion at the terminal stages of the disease was noted in filovirus-infected monkeys by other researchers [Murphy, 1971; Baskerville, 1978]. Lymphoid depletion, an extremely pronounced decrease in the number of lymphocytes, is another striking manifestation of filoviral damage to the immune system in experimental animals. This depletion can be seen in Figure 8-2. Figure 8-2A shows a light microscope photograph of the cortical section of the inguinal lymph node of a green monkey infected with ZEBOV, while Figure 8-2B is the same area in a normal, uninfected monkey. There is an obvious, large decrease in the number of lymphatic follicles and lymphocytes in the infected monkey. Pronounced lymphoid depletion developed from days 3 to 4 in both MARV- and ZEBOV-infected animals. Only a few small lymphoid follicles were encountered in lymphatic tissue at the terminal stages. A lymphoid follicle (nodule) can be seen in Figure 8-3; its center is homogeneous and devoid of any lymphoid cells. The morphological appearance of these nodules (small, homogeneous germinal centers without blast cells) suggests that their function is impaired. The B zones of the lymph nodes were more affected than the T zones; however, the T zones showed no signs of functional activity (B lymphocytes generally produce antibodies and the humoral immunity and T lymphocytes usually attack cells containing viruses and are responsible for cell-mediated immunity). Using morphometric measurements, we observed a 69 percent reduction of the relative volume of the germinal centers of the follicles of the mesenteric lymph nodes within the first 2 days of inoculating green monkeys with ZEBOV. This is consistent with the lymphoid depletion.

Apoptosis was proposed as a mechanism that causes lymphoid depletion and lymphopenia in MARV- and EBOV-infected animals [Geisbert, 2000]. Apoptosis is a very selective mechanism that rapidly kills the chosen cells without altering the surrounding cells. Apoptosis is also responsible for a decrease in the number of plasma cells, as noted by the shrinking of the cells and nuclei.

Figure 8-2. Two light microscope photographs of the cortical portion of the inguinal lymphatic nodes of a green monkey. The photograph in **Figure 8-2A** was made 7 days after inoculation with ZEBOV. The photograph in **Figure 8-2B** was made using tissue from the lymphatic node from a normal, uninfected green monkey. The differences between the photos are the absence of follicles and the paucity of lymphocytes in the infected tissue.

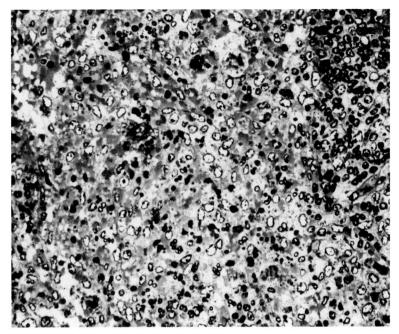

Figure 8-2A

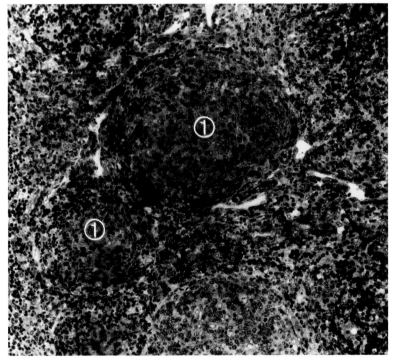

Figure 8-2B

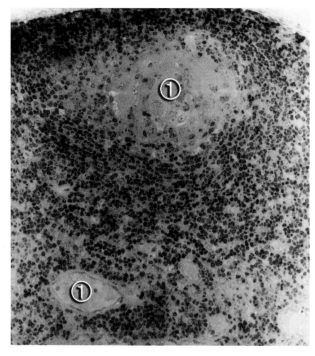

Figure 8-3. Light microscope photographs of a semithin section of the cortical zone of a lymphatic node from an infected monkey. **Figure 8-3A** shows the light homogeneous center of a follicle that is devoid of lymphoid cells. **Figure 8-3B** (duplicate photo of 8-2B) shows the same zone of a lymphatic node in an uninfected monkey; the zone appears much darker.

Figure 8-3A

Legend

Figure 8-3

1. Follicle

See Note on page xiii.

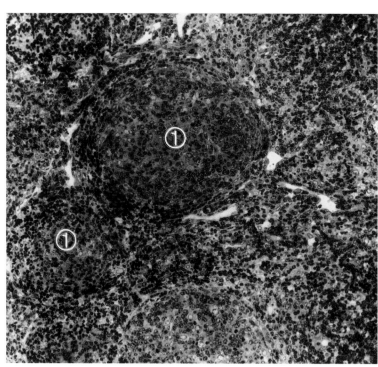

Figure 8-3B

Figure 8-4 shows the apoptosis of lymphocytes and plasma cells from a lymph node of an infected green monkey. Necrosis of the plasma cells was also observed. We did not observe the formation of new plasma cells and consequently, the decrease in plasma cells was not as dramatic as we would have expected. The absence of plasma cell formation is another sign of the impairment of immune functions in fatal filoviral infection. It is particularly interesting that this apoptosis apparently kills immunocompetent cells. This phenomenon reflects one of the events in virus-host

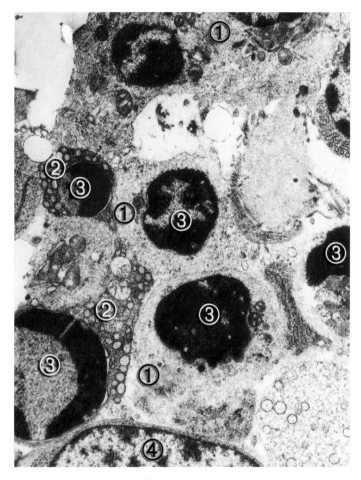

Legend

Figure 8-4

1. Lymphocyte
2. Plasma cell
3. Apoptotic nucleus
4. Unaltered nucleus

See Note on page xiii.

Figure 8-4. Apoptosis of lymphocytes and plasma cells in an infected green monkey's lymphatic node, sampled before death (magnification 8,500). Generally, shrinking or contracting nuclei, often with fragmentation, characterize cells killed by apoptosis. Necrotic cells generally swell and then lyse.

interactions or exploitation by the virus; the virus uses apoptosis to prevent a defensive immune response to preserve the cells that provide its replication. The same pattern also was observed in other viral infections, including influenza [Fujimoto, 2000], swine fever [Summerfield, 1998], and others [Teodoro, 1997]. The involvement of apoptosis in viral pathogenesis probably developed as viruses and hosts co-evolved.

We observed that in filoviral infections, apoptosis occurs in lymphocytes, which do not replicate the viruses, but it is not found in macrophages, which do support viral replication. However, apoptosis of lymphocytes, which can significantly reduce their number, was found only on last days of the disease, after the lymphocyte depletion had been observed. The disappearance of the lymphocytes was most evident at early stages of the infection, and no lymphocyte necroses were observed during the first 4 to 5 days of the infection. So where do the lymphocytes go during filoviral infections? As we discussed in Chapters 5 and 7, we did not observe an increase in the number of lymphocytes in the liver or any other visceral organ as would happen in many virus infections. One of the few tissues we did not study was the bone marrow. Lymphocyte formation begins in the bone marrow, but it is difficult to say to what extent that lymphoid formation in the bone marrow can influence the lymphocytes in peripheral lymphoid organs. Could there be a mechanism whereby changes in the lymphocyte formation affect the lymphocytes in the peripheral lymphoid organs? Another possibility may be an extremely rapid destruction of lymphocytes that leaves no trace of cell debris. We sampled the organs daily, at the same time each morning, so if there is such rapid lymphocyte destruction, this must occur and the cell debris removed in less than 24 hours.

Damage of Macrophages, Stromal, and Dendritic Cells

There were other early changes that also increased over the course of the filoviral disease and were found at all the anatomical lymphatic tissue locations; these changes included swelling and successive destruction of macrophages and stromal cells. These cells were swollen from days 2 to 3 after inoculation with MARV and ZEBOV. Figure 8-5 shows swollen lymphocytes from a MARV-

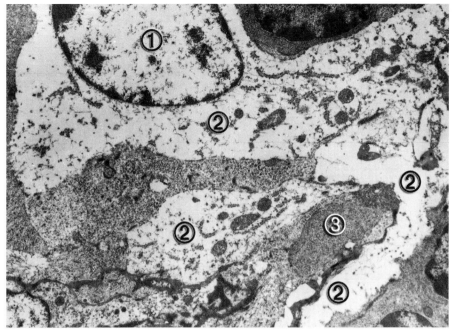

Legend

Figure 8-5

1. Nucleus
2. Cytoplasm
3. Lymphocyte

See Note on page xiii.

Figure 8-5. Swollen stromal (reticular) cell from a MARV-infected green monkey (magnification 7,500). The light swollen reticular cell is visible on the dark background of unaltered lymphocytes in the lymphatic nodes of the infected monkey. These cells were swollen from the first 2 to 3 days post-injection.

infected green monkey. The number of swollen cells increased with the progression of infection. Most macrophages and stromal cells appeared altered at the terminal stages of the disease, despite the fact that only a few of them showed morphological evidence of filoviral reproduction. Widespread alterations in the macrophages and stromal cells of the lymphatic tissue can affect the functions of the immune system; both cell types are involved in the regulation of the immune response [Campbell, 1988; Taub, 1994; Sato, 1995].

Our studies also show that the alteration of macrophages and stromal cells is independent of filoviral infection. This is in contradiction with observations of other authors, who reported massive destruction of filovirus-infected macrophage cells in lymphatic organs [Geisbert, 2000]. This inconsistency may be related to the difference in inoculation dosages. We used small infectious doses in our studies but Geisbert and others used large doses. The large doses result in massive replication of the virus and thus mask some of the pathogenic events. In our studies, the alteration of stromal and macrophage cells is caused by molecular factors, not by virus replication itself.

Macrophages are believed to be crucial for the development of the immune response, and macrophage-dendritic cells are the principal antigen-presenting cells in the development of defensive immune response [Knight, 1988; Steinman, 1991]. The small number of dendritic cells in lymphatic tissue hampers all investigation of these cells in animal lymphatic tissue; therefore, it is not surprising that we failed to find convincing evidence for filoviral reproduction in these cells. We observed viral particles closely associated with protrusions of dendritic cells as shown in Figure 8-6, but we did not observe other indications of viral repro-duction. The dendritic cells also changed morphologically during filoviral infections in monkeys and guinea pigs. Some dendritic cells contained apoptotic nuclei and some contained swollen nuclei. Most dendritic cells were destroyed at the terminal stages of fatal filoviral disease. Although it is clear the dendritic cells are involved, it is not clear how they are involved.

There is an obvious need for a broader approach, including *in vitro* studies, in examining the functions of the dendritic cells in filoviral infection. A broader analysis may enable us to determine the mechanisms of primary filoviral interaction with the host immune system.

Other Pathological Changes

The pathological changes described above are specific to lym-phatic tissue. These changes were found in all the animals irre-spective of the virus, infectious dose, or inoculation route. Furthermore, the alterations in blood vessels in the lymphatic tis-sues were similar to the blood vessel impairments described for the visceral organs in Chapter 7, "Time Course of the Pathologi-cal Changes in Filovirus-Infected Animals." The microcirculatory disturbances appeared on days 2 to 3 post-inoculation, followed by erythrocyte diapedesis and dystrophic changes of the endothelial cells from days 5 and 6 post-inoculation. We described this process

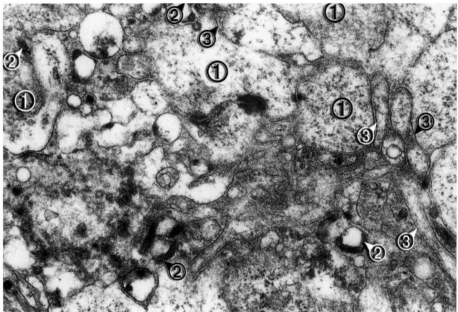

Figure 8-6. Viral particles near the protrusions of dendritic cell (magnification 27,700). The ultrathin section is from the lymphatic node of a ZEBOV-infected green monkey. Although we observed viral particles near the dendritic cells, we did not observe viral replication in these cells (i.e., no viral particles, virions, viral inclusions, or virion budding). We may not have seen this because of the small overall number of dendritic cells.

in Chapter 6, "Blood Disorders in Filoviral Infections." These changes were most pronounced in green and rhesus monkeys infected with ZEBOV. These lymphatic tissues also exhibited fibrin deposits in the blood vessels. When necrotic macrophages were in close proximity to blood vessels, damage to the vessel walls seemed more prominent. This damage was very clear in the lymphatic tissue, in contrast to the unaffected lymphocytes, and this indicates that toxic substances and hydrolases were released from the destroyed macrophages.

Small necrotic foci of lymphatic tissue were observed in filoviral infections in monkeys 2 days before death. Necroses involved all cell types, regardless of whether or not cells were infected. The necroses were probably due to thrombi plugs, which were observed in small vessels. The number and size of such necroses was much greater in animals infected with large doses of MARV and ZEBOV.

The pattern of lesions in lymphatic tissue in different monkey species was the same as in other organs. Accordingly, the lymphatic tissue of green and rhesus monkeys revealed prominent fibrin deposits, whereas the lymph nodes and spleen in baboons showed multiple hemorrhages. These can be seen in Figure 8-7, a light microscope photograph showing hemorrhages in the lymph node of a ZEBOV-infected baboon. There are practically no lymphocytes in the central portion of this photograph. Overall, the

Legend

Figure 8-7

1. Hemorrhage

See Note on page xiii.

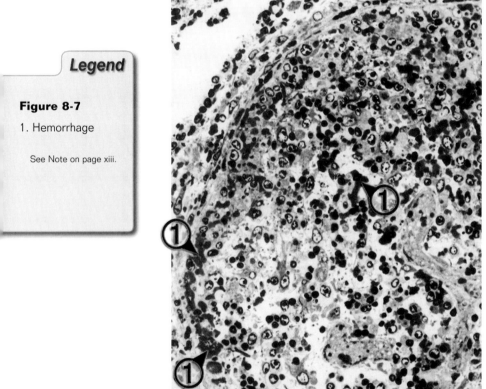

Figure 8-7. Light microscope photograph of severely altered lymphatic node of baboon infected with ZEBOV showing damage of lymphatic tissue and hemorrhages. Note the nearly complete absence of lymphocytes in the central zone of the photo.

pathological changes in lymphoid tissue of filovirus-infected animals characterize a complicated picture in which all the constituents of the lymphatic tissue are altered. In turn, widespread lesions are observed throughout the whole body, supporting the profound nature of the immune system damage.

Lack of Inflammation

The morphologic data show that there is severe damage of the immune system during filoviral diseases, and damage develops in all lymphatic tissue at all anatomical sites. This damage involves all links in the immunity process and affects lymphocyte division and differentiation, macrophages, and dendritic cells. However, there is another feature of immune system impairment that was evident in the visceral organs in fatal filoviral infections: there was a lack of inflammatory reaction to filovirus-infected cells. This was noted in descriptions of the visceral organs in Chapter 7 (leukocytes did not accumulate in the infected tissues) and is common to all fatal MARV and ZEBOV infections in monkeys and guinea pigs. The development of a local inflammatory reaction in the sites of viral reproduction plays a very important role in the disease outcome [Salazar-Mather, 2000]. This reaction is distinct from the destruction of infected cells by effector cells of the immune system, namely specific T-cells, which are destined specifically for the infected cells. The lack of a local inflammatory reaction in filovirus-infected animals is further evidence for the inability of their immune systems to fight the infection.

Immune Responses in Human Filoviral Infections

Recent outbreaks of Ebola hemorrhagic fever in Gabon in 1996 provided an opportunity for more detailed examination of human cases and immune reactions. Examination of the blood samples allows researchers to obtain information about generalized pathological events but cannot provide information about changes in organs. This should be taken into account when analyzing the data. Studies of blood samples obtained during Ebola outbreaks provided very significant information for understanding the pathogenesis of filoviral hemorrhagic fever. Fatal filoviral infections in humans have been shown to be associated with failed humoral immune responses. EBOV-specific immunoglobulin G (IgG) was absent, and very little immunoglobulin M (IgM) was detected in the blood of those patients in whom the infections were fatal. Before death, T-cells disappeared from the blood, indicating severe damage to the cellular immune response [Baize, 1999]. These data correspond to our findings of an incomplete defensive immune response in fatally infected monkeys and guinea pigs. The mechanisms of the blockage of local inflammatory reaction in filoviral infections are not clear but are most likely related to humoral agents.

Examination of ZEBOV-specific antibodies in blood from patients in Gabon, both from fatal infections and from patients who survived, did not provide sufficient information to construct a more satisfactory concept of the role of humoral immune response in filoviral infections [Baize, 1999; Maruyama, 1999]. In contrast, studies of molecular indices of the T-cells from surviving patients showed clear evidence that the infected cells were killed by activated T-cells during the period of recovery from ZEBOV infection [Baize, 1999]. Thus, after the immune response system recovers from the impairment to humoral agents, it performs as needed to kill the filovirus-infected cells.

Possible Mechanisms of Immunity Impairment and Directions of Future Research

As we have discussed, the pattern of damage to immune cells in filovirus-infected animals appears to have several components, with the derangement of immune functions progressing in all the links to other organs. Each derangement can have a strong impact on the immune defense in filovirus-infected subjects. The course of filoviral disease is so rapid that the term "immune deficiency" or "immune suppression" is meaningless; the situation is more adequately described as "immune breakdown." The mechanisms for such an "immune breakdown" are unknown. Understanding these mechanisms would facilitate both treatment and prevention of the filoviral diseases.

Recent publications give a collection of various hypotheses explaining how damage of immunity may be based on the molecular biology of the filoviruses. All these background studies have been performed on model systems and EBOV. Yang [Yang, 1998; Kindzelskii, 2000] proposed that ZEBOV GP interacted with neutrophils and thus interfered with their innate immunity function, but more recent research found no interaction of the GP with neutrophils [Sui, 2000]. EBOV replication is characterized by proteolytic processing of the GP and secretion of sGP. Feldmann and co-authors proposed that proteolytically liberated GPs and perhaps even the proteolytic cleavage itself may be the main molecular factors for EBOV pathogenicity [Feldmann, 1999]. The suggestion seems very interesting, as do other speculations about the GPs' function in filovirus-infected animals. However, what about MARV, which does not produce sGP? MARV causes identical damage to the immune system in experimental animals and, as demonstrated in one of the last outbreaks, has the same impact on humans as EBOV.

Another approach for understanding the immunopathology may well be developed on the background of filoviral genome sequencing. A region of the filoviral genome has been identified that codes for surface glycoprotein. This region showed a high degree of homology with an immunosuppressive motif occurring in retroviruses. It has been suggested that this region of the glycoprotein may provide preferential binding of filoviruses to macrophages participating in the regulation of the immune response [Bukreev, 1993; Volchkov, 1992]. Further studies showed that the immunosuppressive motif is highly conserved and is the single motif in the glycoprotein of all filoviruses [Becker, 1995a]. The exact role this motif plays in filoviral pathogenesis needs detailed examination.

Experiments done at USAMRIID have shown that the fibroblastic reticular cell (FRC) conduit system rapidly transports cytokines to the high endothelial venule (HEV) [Anderson, 1993]. These authors have suggested that EBOV may use the FRC conduit to cross the lymphatic tissues. If the FRC conduit is damaged by filoviral infection, changes in the ability of the immune system will result [Davis, 1997].

Based on our studies, we propose that macrophage infection with the filoviruses leads to a release of mediators that trigger damage to the immune system. These mediators include the tumor necrosis factor (TNF) and interleukins [Bone, 1996; Cook,

1996; Taub, 1994]. The list of macrophage functions is incomplete, but convincing pieces of evidence are filling the gaps. The macrophages are recognized as key cells in the immune system. The macrophage damage we observed during filoviral infections suggests that macrophages may be the main link in a deficient immune defense. Our data provide a basis for further detailed studies of filovirus-induced damage to the immune system.

chapter 9

Conclusions

The electron microscope is a powerful tool that can be used to explore the causes of disease, the structure of viruses, and features that determine their viral pathogenesis. However, the quality and strategy of the experiments are important to how much can be achieved with the electron microscope. While we have used the electron microscope to explore the structure of the filoviruses, study their reproduction, and observe the changes in organs that result, our approach to the experiments has enabled us to develop an understanding of the nature of the infection and resulting disease that goes beyond pictures or curiosities. We have developed a model of filoviral infection and disease that can act as a working hypothesis for other researchers to use, expand upon, and test. We will review the highlights of our studies and previously reported experiments. Then we will present a summary of our model.

Filoviral Infection

Both MARV and EBOV infections begin by infecting macrophages. Regardless of the route of entry, (IP, IV, SC, inhalation, etc.), the filovirus' primary target cell is the macrophage. The infected macrophages (both fixed and circulating) release virions, which are then carried by the blood system to other cells.

Filoviral infection occurs very quickly, when the virus is inoculated directly into the blood and even when inoculated by inhalation. Using MARV and Vero cells, we found the first signs of filoviral replication within 12 hours of inoculation and viral progeny after 21 hours.

We also explored the quality of filoviral replications and the time that the virions were produced. In our studies of MARV and ZEBOV in Vero cells, we noted that the rod-shaped virions are those that appear to reproduce most effectively. In Vero cells, the viral budding in MARV starts at about 20 hours post-inoculation and continues over about 36 hours (viral replication cycle). We did not determine the replication cycle for ZEBOV but we expect it to be similar. As the course of the infection progresses, the rod-shaped virions become less dominant and account for smaller percentages of the observed virions both in the cultured cells and in ZEBOV-infected animals. What is the role of these polymorphic virions? Do they cause more or less effects in organisms? At this point, we can only raise the questions. We have no way yet of measuring or determining this.

Filoviral infections are rapid in animals and appear to be related to both dose and inoculation routes. Using various doses of MARV or ZEBOV, filoviruses have been found in the blood 2–72 hours after inhalation (MARV—guinea pig; ZEBOV—rhesus monkey), and 4 days after subcutaneous inoculation (ZEBOV—baboon). The filovirus is a very efficient and rapid infectious agent. Other studies have shown that only one viral particle is sufficient to cause filoviral infection and subsequent disease, which presents a challenge to any experiments examining the viral pathogenesis. In order to identify the target cells and subsequent dissemination of viral progeny for our experiments, we needed to use low doses of filovirus (2–5 LD_{50}), and we needed to examine organs and collect samples daily.

Using the low infectious doses, we found viremia within hours of inoculation. We also found that the secondary target cells are hepatocytes and then adrenal cortical cells. Whereas using large infectious doses, other researchers identified endothelial and fibroblast cells as target cells. In our low infectious dose experiments, we found that these cells were only rarely infected, and then only at the terminal stages. We also noted that only the endothelial cells in capillaries were likely to be infected. The larger infectious doses overwhelm the host early in the infection and obscure the development of the disease in the various organs and cells.

Infections in the lungs of animals are significant if inhalation is an important mode of viral transmission. We noted that in some monkey species infected with ZEBOV, and guinea pigs infected with MARV, rare alveolar epithelial cells and ciliated cells, as well as alveolar macrophages were infected. Usually, this infection occurred in areas of the lungs where there was severe lung tissue damage. Thus, aerosol transmission of filoviruses, while not a very effective or efficient process, can occur and should not be neglected.

Lymphocytes and neutrophils were never infected. This is significant because some of the disturbances we noted in the immune system and even the blood system cannot be due to viral infections of the lymphocytes or neutrophils. We also did not find filoviral infections in nerve cells, smooth or striated muscle cells, epithelial cells of the intestines or stomach, pancreatic exocrine cells, or salivary glands.

Disease and Pathology

Although it is important to find the target cells and dissemination pathways, filoviral diseases are not characterized only by changes in the cells in which the filoviruses replicate. The most dramatic characteristics of Ebola and Marburg fevers are the widespread hemorrhages in many of the organs, especially the liver and spleen. The first thoughts for hemorrhages are changes in the blood vessel walls and the endothelial cells. Since we only rarely found infected endothelial cells, there must be other factors at work. In fact, we found that changes in the blood supply or micro-circulation system were involved in all the prominent pathological changes of the visceral organs.

The organs most affected by filoviral infection are the spleen, adrenals, kidneys, and bone marrow. The changes in these organs are predominantly due to changes or damage to the microcirculation system. Changes in the microcirculation system begin within the first days of infection. EBOV infections result in more extensive lesions and blood system damage than MARV infections. EBOV infections often result in DIC, whereas MARV infections, although producing severe damage to blood circulation, including hemorrhages, do not manifest all the characteristics of DIC. We differentiate DIC morphologically as characterized by extensive fibrin deposits and thrombi throughout all the organs. MARV infections were characterized by having fibrin deposits only in the necrotic areas where fibrin masses were produced by plasma exudates. Even in ZEBOV infections in monkeys there were species-related differences in circulation damage and not every animal developed DIC. This difference between pathologies in Ebola and Marburg disease, we propose, may be due to the role of EBOV's sGP, which is released from the infected cell. This is the only viral protein different between the two filoviruses.

Microcirculation system damage is responsible for most of the pathology in most of the organs. However, in some organs, such as the adrenals, disruption of function appears as a result of virus infection and not as a hemostatic disorder. We attribute the micro-circulation damage to changes in the cytokine profile that are triggered by the infection of monocytes/macrophages. These changes account for variations in blood vessel permeability, as well as other related functions. The microcirculation system damage is responsible for most of the pathology in most of the organs. This damage starts early in the disease and is not a result of infections in the endothelial cells of the blood vessel walls. This is consistent with the release of mediators from infected macrophages.

We saw pronounced damage in the alveolar capillaries of the lungs that was not due to infected endothelial cells. This micro-circulation system damage undoubtedly was caused by the infected macrophages' cytokine profile changes and indicates that the oxygen supply for the animal is critically damaged.

Inflammatory Response

A notable observation in examining the pathologies of filoviral infections was the absence of inflammation in the organs. We did not see an increase in lymphocytes or swelling of cells and tissues, which indicates that the immune system is impaired. The macrophage, which normally manages immune reactions and ingests infected cells and foreign material as part of the immune response to infection, is itself the target of the infection and the normal release of cell mediators and cytokines is disrupted. The infected macrophage does release mediators that damage the immune system, such as tumor necrosis factor (TNF) and interleukins. This immune system damage is responsible for the devastating effects of disease.

We examined the lymphatic system, and noted that lymphocyte mitosis and differentiation were no longer occurring. Indeed, lymphoid depletion became obvious. Macrophages that were not infected often were altered, shortly after inoculation. These macrophages and stromal cells appeared swollen. We attribute the lymphoid depletion partly to apoptosis and note that we saw evidence of apoptosis (contracting nuclei) at the last stages of the disease. Lymphoid depletion actually occurs earlier in the course of the disease, but exactly where the lymphocytes go or how quickly they are destroyed is not clear.

Animal Models for Filoviral Studies

There are different approaches to choosing animals for experimental studies. Sometimes it is enough for the study that an animal develops a fatal infection after viral inoculation. Certainly in the initial stages of investigating a disease this is appropriate. However, investigations of the mechanisms of pathogenesis need more careful and considered choices. Our studies can provide a guide for how to select the best animal species depending on the goal of the experiment. For example, guinea pigs are a good choice if the focus of the investigation is on the mechanisms of changes in the immune system during MARV infections. Green monkeys are appropriate for studies of pathogenesis and damage of immunity in MARV infection. Comparative studies of MARV infection in various monkey species should be performed to understand species-specific features of the infection and to find a species in which the disease development is more similar to Marburg hemorrhagic fever in humans.

Our data to date suggest that the baboon may be the closest model to humans for investigating various aspects of ZEBOV infection, including damage to the blood. Other monkey species (green, cynomolgus, and rhesus monkeys) showed different patterns of damage in the blood system. (Our studies at Vector are the only reported ZEBOV studies using baboons.) However, these differences in disease patterns may be exploited to investigate the detailed mechanisms of how the blood system damage develops and which viral or host factors are responsible for development of different hemostatic injuries. On the other hand, even the use of baboons as a model for human infection is complicated by the variety of responses in both baboons and humans and the large number of unknowns in terms of dose, routes of infection, and variations in genetic susceptibility.

What Directly Causes Rapid Death in Filoviral Infections?

As a rule, filovirus-infected animals die within 6 to 10 days after inoculation. The direct cause of death in filovirus-infected humans and experimental animals has not been established. MARV- and EBOV-infected animals die after a brief terminal shock. None of the damage to the visceral organs was sufficient to have been directly responsible for lethality [Fisher-Hoch, 1985; Peters, 1996]. However, we observed damage to the blood system in the lung sections of all our experimental animals and this damage was widespread. Our ultrastructure examinations with the electron microscope revealed neutrophil accumulation and multiple thromboses of the alveolar capillaries at the terminal stages of infection. The neutrophils themselves have been implicated as the cause of alveolar thrombosis mediated by release of oxygen intermediates [Leaver, 1995; Mayanskiy, 1995; Murohara, 1994; Risberg, 1991; Smith, 1994; Thelen, 1993].

The significance of neutrophils in filoviral infections demands closer scrutiny. Neutrophils act as the major triggers in the development of acute respiratory distress syndrome (ARDS) and severe lung damage, which leads to death in many pathological processes [Leaver, 1995; Murohara, 1994; Smith, 1994]. The humoral agents released from neutrophils, including TNF, induce a release of active mediators from the neutrophils. The TNF stimulates neutrophil aggregation, degranulation, and respiratory burst, all of which profoundly damage blood vessels and tissue [Barnard, 1995; Downey, 1995; Movat, 1987; Salyer, 1990; Shalaby, 1985]. ARDS was observed in humans in Lassa hemorrhagic fever and in guinea pigs inoculated with *Pichinde* virus, both members of the *Arenaviridae* family [Schaeffer, 1993].

Our studies established that the macrophages, the main producers of TNF, are involved in pathogenic reactions from the first stages of filoviral infections. We suggest that macrophages affected by filoviruses release inflammatory mediators, including the TNF that impairs lung microcirculation. In fact, an increase in serum TNF level was reported during Marburg virus infection of guinea pigs and monkeys [Ignatiev, 1994; Ignatiev, 1995].

Accordingly, we propose that the accumulation and degranulation of neutrophils in alveolar capillaries may induce the acute respiratory distress syndrome that is usually lethal. The high levels of TNF that may be produced by macrophages may contribute to development of ARDS by inducing the release of active oxygen intermediaries from neutrophils.

Crucial Role of the Macrophages

Macrophages are the primary targets for filoviruses, and macrophages are directly involved in the function of the blood system and immunity. Thus, their role in development of filoviral infection is critical. Undoubtedly, infection of the macrophages with MARV and EBOV alters their functions and affects the whole macrophage system. The release of various mediators by infected and uninfected macrophages also affects the blood system. These mediators may influence many, if not all, physiological functions in the organism. Distribution of the mediators by blood and lymph involves all the organs and tissues in a pathological process. Macrophages, infected by filoviruses, appear to induce a cascade of pathological reactions by liberating various mediators. Some of these may be the interleukins (e.g., IL-1 and IL-6), gamma-interferon, and TNF-alpha. These substances are known to impair immunity, microcirculation, blood clotting, vessel permeability, and many other processes [Bendtzen, 1988; Heller,

1994; Le, 1989]. The levels of these mediators have been correlated with the severity of disease in humans caused by Dengue virus [Hober, 1993; Kuno, 1994; Yang, 1995]. However, it is easy to suggest that these mediators may be involved, but it is very difficult to evaluate exactly which mediators operate in infected organisms and which cells produce these mediators. It is difficult to determine the origin of each substance in the blood. So, while it is easy to state that filoviral infection of macrophages is the critical pathogenic event, it is not easy to establish this experimentally.

Systemic Aspects of Fatal EBOV and MARV Infections

We have determined, using our experiments and other internationally reported findings, that the disease developing from filoviral infection largely corresponds to an acute intravascular inflammation that develops on a background where the immune defense system is functionally compromised. Most of the principal events in the disease development are related to the blood system: primary virus reproduction in macrophages, alteration of microcirculation, virus dissemination, distribution of mediators, changes in blood cell counts, accumulation of neutrophils, damage to the blood system, and finally, lesions in endothelial cells at the terminal stages of disease. As we have noted, these alterations in blood tissue are shown in the pathology of all the affected organs and represent systemic damage to the organism. Recent studies of asymptomatic, non-fatal, and fatal EBOV infections in humans have been performed using immunoassays and PCR to detect various biologically active substances and indices of the immune system. These studies were in agreement that an effective inflammatory response was needed to control the replication of filoviruses and prevent the development of symptoms. In particular, the researchers noted the presence of three cytokines in the asymptomatic patients that were absent in symptomatic patients: IL-1ß, IL-6, and TNF [Leroy, 2000]. These three cytokines can be produced by macrophages, but other cells and factors can also contribute to the presence of these cytokines in the blood. Our data are not inconsistent with this recent study. In fact, both our studies and Leroy's work suggest that the role of cytokines and inflammatory reactions in filoviral infections and disease needs to be further explored.

Our research in filoviruses relied heavily on the use of electron microscopy to detect the filoviruses, look for their replication in cells, and explore the pathology of the organs. Our experiments stressing the very small infectious doses of filoviruses were critical in determining the role of macrophages as the primary target. Such experiments are essential in eliciting the role of the immune defenses in pathogenesis. These time course experiments also revealed that although other cells, in particular the endothelial cells and fibroblasts, did support filoviral replication, they did so only at the terminal stages of the disease and probably did not contribute significantly to the impairment of the immune system functions. The infected macrophages appear to impair the immune system by the release of factors such as TNF and inter-leukins. Our experiments also led us to propose that damage to the blood system in the lungs, perhaps with acute respiratory dis-tress, was the cause of death in all the animals. Liver infection, while often severe, was not the dominant, common disruption in the organisms that necessarily resulted in death, and in fact, we observed that death occasionally occurred without infection of the hepatocytes. Our work has indicated that further research on the role of the macrophages in releasing factors that affect the inflam-matory reactions will be required to develop effective treatments to filoviral infections. The systemic involvement of the factors filovirus-infected macrophages release may well lead to treatments for both Ebola and Marburg hemorrhagic fevers. In any case, the role these factors play in the disease is critical to understanding filoviral infection and perhaps other viruses that attack macrophages.

References

Akira, S., Taga, T., and Kishimoto, T. (1993) Interleukin-6 in biology and medicine. *Adv. Immunol.* **54** (1), 1–5.

Almeida, J.D., Waterson, A.P., and Simpson, D.J.H. (1971) *Morphology and Morphogenesis of the Marburg Agent, Marburg Virus Disease* (Eds G.A. Martini and R. Siegert). Berlin: Springer-Verlag, 84–97.

Anderson, A.O. and Shaw, S. (1993) T cell adhesion to endothelium: the FRC conduit system and other anatomic and molecular features which facilitate the adhesion cascade in lymph node. *Semin. Immunol.* **5** (4), 271–282.

Baize, S., Leroy, E.M., Georges-Courbout, M.C., Capron, M., Lansoud-Soukate, J., Debre, P., Fisher-Hoch, S.P., McCormick, J.B., and Georges, A.J. (1999) Defective humoral responses and extensive intravascular apoptosis are associated with fatal outcome in Ebola virus-infected patients. *Nat. Med.* **5** (4), 423–426.

Barlowe, C., Orci, L., Yeung, T., Hosobuchi, M., Hamamoto, S., Salama, N., Rexach, M.F., Ravazzola, M., Amherdt, M., and Schekman, R. (1994) COPII: a membrane coat formed by Sec proteins that drive vesicle budding from the endoplasmic reticulum. *Cell.* **77** (6), 895–907.

Barnard, J.W., Biro, M.G., Lo, S.K., Ohno, S., Carozza, M.A., Moyle, M., Soule, H.R., and Malik, A.B. (1995) Neutrophil inhibitory factor prevents neutrophil-dependent lung injury. *J. Immunol.* **155** (10), 4876–4881.

Baskerville, A., Bowen, E.T., Platt, G.S., McArdell, L.B., and Simpson, D.I. (1978) The pathology of experimental Ebola virus infection in monkeys. *J. Pathol.* **125** (3), 131–138.

Baskerville, A., Fisher-Hoch, S.P., Neild, G.H., and Dowsett, A.B. (1985) Ultrastructural pathology of experimental Ebola haemorrhagic fever virus infection. *J. Pathol.* **147** (3), 199–209.

Becker, S., Spiess, M., Klenk, H.D. (1995) The asialoglycoprotein receptor is a potential liver-specific receptor for Marburg virus. *J. Gen. Virol.* **76** (Pt 2), 393–399.

Becker, Y. (1995a) Retrovirus and filovirus "immunosuppressive motif" and the evolution of virus pathogenicity in HIV-1, HIV-2, and Ebola viruses. *Virus Genes.* **11** (2–3), 191–195.

Bendtzen, K. (1988) Interleukin-1, interleukin-6 and tumor necrosis factor in infection, inflammation and immunity. *Immunol. Lett.* **19** (3), 183–191.

Bertherat, E., Talarmin, A., Zeller, H. (1999) Democratic Republic of the Congo: between civil war and the Marburg virus. International Committee of Technical and Scientific Coordination of the Durba Epidemic. *Med. Trop.* **59** (2), 201–204 (in French).

Biel, S.S. and Gelderblom, H.R. (1999) Diagnostic electron microscopy is still a timely and rewarding method. *J. Clin. Virol.* 1999 **13** (1–2), 105–119.

Bogdan, C. and Nathan, C. (1993) Modulation of macrophage function by transforming growth factor beta, interleukin-4, and interleukin-10. *Ann. N.Y. Acad. Sci.* **685**, 713–717.

Bone, R.C. (1996) Toward a theory regarding the pathogenesis of the systemic inflammatory response syndrome: what we do and do not know about cytokine regulation. *Crit. Care Med.* **24** (1), 163–172.

Bouree, P. and Bergmann, J.F. (1983) Ebola virus infection in man: a serological and epidemiological survey in the Cameroons. *Am. J. Trop. Med. Hyg.* **32** (6), 1465–1466.

Bowen, E.T., Lloyd, G., Harris, W.J., Platt, G.S., Baskerville, A., and Vella, E.E. (1977) Viral haemorrhagic fever in southern Sudan and northern Zaire. Preliminary studies on the aetiological agent. *Lancet.* **1** (8011), 571–573.

Bray, M., Hatfill, S., Hensley, L., and Huggins, J.W. (2001) Haematological, biochemical and coagulation changes in mice, guinea-pigs and monkeys infected with a mouse-adapted variant of Ebola Zaire virus. *J. Comp. Path.* **125** (4), 243–253.

Bukreyev, A.A., Volchkov, V.E., Blinov, V.M., and Netesov, S.V. (1993) The GP-protein of Marburg virus contains the region similar to the "immunosuppressive domain" of oncogenic retrovirus P15E proteins. *FEBS Lett.* **323** (1–2), 183–187.

Bukreyev, A.A., Volchkov, V.E., Blinov, V.M., Dryga, S.A., and Netesov, S.V. (1995) The complete nucleotide sequence of the Popp (1967) strain of Marburg virus: a comparison with the Musoke (1980) strain. *Arch. Virol.* **140** (9), 1589–1600.

Campbell, A.D., and Wicha, M.S. (1988) Extracellular matrix and the hematopoetic microenvironment. *J. Lab. Clin. Med.* **112** (2), 140–146.

Campetella, O.E., Sanchez, A., and Giovaniello, O.A. (1988) In vivo Junin virus-mouse macrophage interaction. *Acta Virol.* **32** (3), 198–206.

Centers for Disease Control and Prevention. (1990) CDC Update: Filovirus Infection Associated with Contact with Nonhuman Primates or Their Tissues. *MMWR.* **39** (24), 404.

Chan, S.Y., Speck, R.F., Ma, M.C., and Goldsmith, M.A. (2000) Distinct mechanisms of entry by envelope glycoproteins of Marburg and Ebola (Zaire) viruses. *J. Virol.* **74** (10), 4933–4937.

Chan, S.Y., Empig, C.J., Welte, F.J., Speck, R.F., Schmaljohn, A., Kreisberg, J.F., and Goldsmith, M.A. (2001) Folate receptor-alpha is a cofactor for cellular entry by Marburg and Ebola viruses. *Cell.* **106** (1), 117–126.

Chain, B.M., Kaye, P.M., and Shaw, M.A. (1988) The biochemistry and cell biology of antigen processing. *Immunol. Rev.* **106**, 33–58.

Chermashentsev, V.M., Zhukov, V.A., Maryasov, A.G., and Safatov, A.S. (1993) Theoretical approaches to the evaluation of antiviral drug effectiveness. *Vestn. Ross. Akad. Med. Nauk.* (9), 3–7.

Chua, K.G., Koh, C.L., Hoopi, P.S., Wee, K.F., Khong, J.H., Chua, B.H., Chan, Y.P., Lim, M.E., Lam, S.K. (2002) Isolation of Nipah virus from Malaysian Island flying-foxes. *Microbes Infect.* **4** (2), 145–151.

Cook, D.N. (1996) The role of MIP-1 alpha in inflammation and hematopoiesis. *J. Leukoc. Biol.* **59** (1), 61–66.

Connolly, B.M., Steele, K.E., Davis, K.J., Geisbert, T.W., Kell, W.M., Jaax, N.K., and Jahrling, P.B. (1999) Pathogenesis of experimental Ebola virus infection in guinea pigs. *J. Infect. Dis.* **179** (Suppl. 1), S203–S217.

Cosgriff, T.M. (1989)Viruses and hemostasis. *Rev. Infec. Dis.* **11** (Suppl. 4), S672–S688.

Cresswell, P. (1994) Assembly, transport, and function of MHC class II molecules. *Annu. Rev. Immunol.* **12**, 259–293.

Davis, K.J., Anderson, A.O., Geisbert, T.W., Steele, K.E., Geisbert, J.B., Vogel, P.,

Connolly, B.M., Huggins, J.W., Jahrling, P.B., and Jaax, N.K. (1997) Pathology of experimental Ebola virus infection in African green monkeys. Involvement of fibroblastic reticular cells. *Arch. Pathol. Lab. Med.* **121** (8), 805–819.

Dimmock, N.J. (1982) Review article initial stages in infection with animal viruses. *J. Gen. Virol.* **59** (Pt 1), 1–22.

Downey, G.P., Fialkow, L., and Fukushima, T. (1995) Initial interaction of leukocytes within the microvasculature: deformability, adhesion, and transmigration. *New Horiz.* **3** (2) 219–228.

Draper, C.C. (1977) Hemorrhagic fever in Africa due to Marburg-Ebola viruses. *Disasters*. **1** (4), 309–315.

Ellis, D.S., Simpson, I.H., Francis, D.P., Knobloch, J., Bowen, E.T., Lolok, P., and Deng, I.M. (1978) Ultrastructure of Ebola virus particles in human liver. *J. Clin. Pathol.* **31** (2), 201–208.

Ellis, D.S., Bowen, E.T., Simpson, D.I., and Stamford, S. (1978a) Ebola virus: a comparison, at ultrastructural level, of the behaviour of the Sudan and Zaire strains in monkeys. *Br. J. Exp. Pathol.* **59** (6), 584–593.

Ellis, D.S., Stamford, S., Lloyd, G., Bowen, E.T., Platt, G.S., Way, H., and Simpson, D.I. (1979) Ebola and Marburg viruses: I. Some ultrastructural differences between strains when grown in Vero cells. *J. Med. Virol.* **4** (3), 201–211.

Ellis, D.S., Stamford, S., Tovey, D.G., Lloyd G., Bowen, E.T., Platt, G.S., Way, H., and Simpson, D.I. (1979a) Ebola and Marburg viruses: II. Their development within Vero cells and the extracellular formation of branched and torus forms. *J. Med. Virol.* **4** (3), 213–225.

Empig C.J. and Goldsmith, M.A. (2002). Association of the caveola vesicular system with cellular entry by filoviruses. *J. Virol.* **76** (10), 5266–70.

Esmon, C.T. (1999) Possible involvement of cytokines in diffuse intravascular coagulation and thrombosis. *Best Pract. Res. Clin. Haematol.* **12** (3), 343–359.

Feldmann, H., Will, C., Schikore, M., Slenczka, W., Klenk, H.D. (1991) Glycosylation and oligomerization of the spike protein of Marburg virus. *Virology*. **182** (1), 353–356.

Feldmann, H., Mühlberger, E., Randolf, A., Will, C., Kiley, M.P., Sanchez, A., and Klenk, H.D. (1992) Marburg virus, a filovirus: messenger RNAs, gene order, and regulatory elements of the replication cycle. *Virus Res.* **24** (1), 1–19.

Feldmann, H., Bugany, H., Mahner, F., Klenk, H.-D., Drenckhanh, D., and Schnittler, H.-J. (1994) Virus-induced endothelial leakage by infected macrophages. *FASEB J.* **8** (5), A756.

Feldmann, H., Nichol, S.T., Klenk, H.-D., Peters, C.J., and Sanchez, A. (1994a) Characterization of filoviruses based on differences in structure and antigenecity of the virion glycoprotein. *Virology.* **199** (2), 469–473.

Feldmann, H., Bugany, H., Mahner, F., Klenk, H.D., Drenckhahn, D., and Schnittler, H.J. (1996) Filovirus-induced endothelial leakage triggered by infected monocytes/macrophages. *J. Virol.* **70** (4), 2208–2214.

Feldmann, H. and Klenk, H.D. (1996a) Marburg and Ebola viruses. *Adv. Virus Res.* **47**, 1–52.

Feldmann, H., Volchkov, V.E., Volchkova, V.A., and Klenk, H.D. (1999) The glycoproteins of Marburg and Ebola viruses and their potential roles in pathogenesis. *Arch. Virol. Suppl.* **15**, 159–169.

Feldmann, H. and Kiley, M.P. (1999a) Classification, structure, and replication of filoviruses. *Curr. Top. Microbiol. Immunol.* **235**, 1–21.

Feldmann, H., Volchkov, V.E., Volchkova, V.A., Ströher, U., and Klenk, H.D. (2001) Biosynthesis and role of filoviral glycoproteins. *J. Gen. Virol.* **82** (Pt 12), 2839–2848

Fisher-Hoch, S.P., Platt, G.S., Neild, G.H., Southee, T., Baskerville, A., Raymond, R.T., Lloyd, G., and Simpson, D.I. (1985) Pathophysiology of shock and hemorrhage in fulminating viral infection (Ebola). *J. Infect. Dis.* **152** (5) 887–894.

Fisher-Hoch, S.P., Brammer, T.L., Trappier, S.G., Hutwagner, L.C., Farrar, B.B., Ruo, S.L., Brown, B.G., Hermann, L.M., Perez-Oronoz, G.I., Goldsmith, C.S., et al. (1992) Pathogenic potential of filoviruses: role of geographic origin of primate host and virus strain. *J. Infect. Dis.* **166** (4), 753–763.

Formenty, P., Hatz, C., LeGuenno, B., Stoll, A., Rogenmoser, P., and Widmer, A. (1999) Human infection due to Ebola virus, subtype Cote d'Ivoire: clinical and biological presentation. *J. Infect. Dis.* **179** (Suppl. 1), S48–S53.

Formenty, P., Boesch, C., Wyers, M., Steiner, C., Donati, F., Dind, F., Walker, F., and LeGuenno, B. (1999a) Ebola virus outbreak among wild chimpanzees living in a rain forest of Cote d'Ivoire. *J. Infect. Dis.* **179** (Suppl 1), S120–S126.

Fujimoto, I., Pan, J., Takizawa, T., and Nakanishi, Y. (2000) Virus clearance through apoptosis-dependent phagocytosis of influenza A virus-infected cells by macrophages. *J. Virol.* **74** (7), 3399–3403.

Fujishima, S. and Aikawa, N. (1995) Neutrophil-mediated tissue injury and its modulation. *Intensive Care Med.* **21** (3), 277–285.

Gear, J.S., Cassel, G.A., Gear, A.J., et al. (1975) Outbreak of Marburg virus disease in Johannesburg. *Br. Med. J.* **4** (5995) 489–493.

Geisbert, T.W., Jahrling, P.B., Hanes, M.A., and Zack, P.M. (1992) Association of Ebola-related Reston virus particles and antigen with tissue lesions of monkeys imported to the United States. *J. Comp. Path.* **106** (2), 137–152.

Geisbert, T.W. and Jahrling, P.B. (1995) Differentiation of filoviruses by electron microscopy. *Virus Res.* **39** (2–3), 129–150.

Geisbert, T.W., and Jaax, N.K. (1998) Marburg hemorrhagic fever: report of a case studied by immunohistochemistry and electron microscopy. *Ultrastruct. Pathol.* **22** (1), 3–17.

Geisbert, T.W., Hensley, L.E., Gibb, T.R., Steele, K.E., Jaax, N.K., and Jahrling, P.B. (2000) Apoptosis induced in vitro and in vivo during infection by Ebola and Marburg viruses. *Lab Invest.* **80** (2), 171–186.

Georges, A.J., Renaut, A.A., Bertherat, E., Baize, S., Leroy, E., LeGuenno, B., Lepage, J., Amblard, J., Edzang, S., and Georges-Courbot, M.C. (1996) Recent Ebola virus outbreaks in Gabon from 1994 to 1996: epidemiologic and control issues (Ebola virus research 4–7 Sept 1996, Antwerp, Belgium). *Abstr. Intern. Coll.* p. 47.

Georges, A.J, Leroy, E.M., Renaut, A.A., Benissan, C.T., Nabias, R.J., Ngoc, M.T., Obiang, P.I., Lepage, J.P, Bertherat, E.J., Benoni, D.D., Wickings, E.J., Amblard, J.P., Lansourd-Soukate, J.M., Milleliri, J.M., Baize, S., and Georges-Courbot, M.C. (1999) Ebola hemorrhagic fever outbreaks in Gabon, 1994-1997: epidemiological and health control issues. *J. Infect. Dis.* **179** (Suppl. 1), S65–S75.

Gibb, T. R., Bray, M., Geisbert, T.W., Steele, K.E., Kell, W.M., Davis, K.J., and Jaax, N.K. (2001) Pathogenesis of experimental Ebola Zaire virus infection in BALB/c mice. *J. Comp. Path.* **125** (4), 233–242.

Gonzalez, J.P., Nakoune, E., Slenczka, W., Vidal, P., and Morvan, J.M. (2000) Ebola and Marburg virus antibody prevalence in selected populations of the Central African Republic. *Microbes Infect.* **2** (1), 39–44.

Gupta, M., Mahanty, S., Ahmed, R., and Rollin, P.E. (2001) Monocyte-derived human macrophages and peripheral blood mononuclear cells infected with ebola virus secrete MIP-1 alpha and TNF-alpha and inhibit poly-IC-induced IFN-alpha in vitro. *Virology.* **284** (1), 20–25.

Haass, R., and Maass, G. (1971) Experimental infection of monkeys with the Marburg virus. Marburg Virus Disease (Eds G.A. Martini and R. Siegert), pp. 136–143. Berlin: Springer-Verlag.

Hamilton, P.J., Stalker, A.L., and Douglas, A.S. (1978) Disseminated intravascular coagulation: a review. *J. Clin. Pathol.* **31** (7), 609–619.

Harcourt, B.H., Sanchez, A., and Offermann, M.K. (1998) Ebola virus inhibits induction of genes by double-stranded RNA in endothelial cells. *Virology*. **252** (1), 179–188.

Harcourt, B.H., Sanchez, A., and Offermann, M.K. (1999) Ebola virus selectively inhibits responses to interferons, but not to interleukin-1beta, in endothelial cells. *J. Virol.* **73** (4), 3491–3496.

Hayes, C.G., Burans, J.P., Ksiazek, T.G., et al. (1992) Outbreak of fatal illness among captive macaques in the Philippines caused by an Ebola-related filovirus. *Am. J. Trop. Med. Hyg.* **46** (6), 664–671

Heller, R.A. and Kronke, M. (1994) Tumor necrosis factor receptor-mediated signaling pathways. *J. Cell Biol.* **126** (1), 5–9.

Hevey, M., Negley, D., Geisbert, J., Jahrling, P., and Schmaljohn, A. (1997) Antigenicity and vaccine potential of Marburg virus glycoprotein expressed by baculovirus recombinants. *Virology*. **239** (1), 206–216.

Hober, D., Poli, L., Roblin, B., Gestas, P., Chungue, E., Granic, G., Imbert, P., et al. (1993) Serum levels of tumor necrosis factor-alpha (TNF-alpha), interleukin-6 (IL-6), and interleukin-1 beta (IL-1 beta) in dengue-infected patients. *Am. J. Trop. Med. Hyg.* **48** (3), 324–331.

Hopkins, C.R. (1983) The importance of the endosome in intracellular traffic. *Nature*. **304** (5928), 684–685.

Ignatiev, G.M., Agafonov, A.P., Prosorovskii, N.S., Shukova, N.A., Kashentseva, E.A., and Vorobeva, M.S. (1994) Immunological measurements in Marburg virus infected guinea pigs. *Voprosi Virusologii*. (4), 169–171.

Ignatiev, G.M., Streltsova, M.A., Agafonov, A.P., and Kashentseva, E.A. (1995) Mechanisms of protective immune response in Marburg virus infected monkeys. *Voprosi Virusologii*. (3), 109–112.

Ikegami, T., Calaor, A.B., Miranda, M.E., Niikura, M., Saijo, M., Kurane, I., Yoshikawa, Y., and Morikawa, S. (2001) Genome structure of Ebola virus subtype Reston: differences among Ebola subtypes. Brief Report. *Arch. Virol.* **146** (10), 2021–2027.

International Committee of Taxonomy of Viruses. *ICTVdB: The Universal Virus Database of the International Committee on Taxonomy of Viruses*. <http://www.ncbi.nlm.nih.gov/ICTVdb/Ictv/index.htm> (updated 28 June 2002).

Isaacson, M. (2001) Viral hemorrhagic fever hazards for travelers in Africa. *Clin. Infect. Dis.* **33** (10), 1707–1712.

Jaax, N.K., Davis, K.J., Geisbert, T.J., et al. (1996) Lethal experimental infection of rhesus monkeys with Ebola-Zaire (Mayinga) virus by the oral and conjunctival route of exposure. *Arch. Pathol. Lab. Med.* **120** (2), 140–155.

Jacobson, S. and Biddson, W.E. (1986) Virus-specific HLA class II-restricted cytotoxic cells. *Concepts in viral pathogenesis II.* Springer-Verlag N.Y. Inc., 187–192.

Jahrling, P.B., Geisbert, T.W., Dalgard, D.W., Johnson, E.D., Ksiazek, T.G., Hall, W.C., and Peters, C.J. (1990) Preliminary report: isolation of Ebola virus from monkeys imported to USA. *Lancet.* **335** (8688), 502–505.

Jahrling, P.B., Geisbert, T.W., Geisbert, J.B., Swearengen, J.R., Bray, M., Jaax, N.K., Huggins, J.W., LeDuc, J.W., and Peters, C.J. (1999) Evaluation of Immune Globulin and Recombinant Interferon –a2b for Treatment of Experimental Ebola Virus Infections. *J. Infect. Dis.* **179** (Suppl. 1), S224–S234.

Janoff, A. and Carp, H. (1982) Proteases, antiproteases, and oxidants: pathways of tissue injury during inflammation. *Monogr. Pathol.* (23), 62–82.

Johnson, E., Jaax, N., White, J., and Jahrling, P. (1995) Lethal experimental infections of rhesus monkeys by aerosolized Ebola virus. *Int. J. Exper. Pathol.* **76** (4), 227–236.

Kachko, A.V., Cheusova, T.B., Sorokin, A.V., Kazachinskaia, E.I., Cheshenko, I.O., Belanov, E.F., Bukreev, A.A., Ivanova, A.V., Razumov, I.A., Riabchikova, E.I., and Netesov S.V. (2001) Comparative study of the morphology and antigenic properties of recombinant analogs of a Marburg virus nucleoprotein. *Molecular Biology (Mosk).* **35** (3), 492–499. Russian.

Kiley, M.P., Bowen, E.T., Eddy, G.A., Isaacson, M., Johnson, K.M., McCormick, J.B., Murphy, F.A., Pattyn, S.R., Peters, D., Prozesky, O.W., Regnery, R.L., Simpson, D.I., Slenczka, W., Sureau, P., van der Groen, G., Webb, P.A., and Wulff, H. (1982) Filoviridae: a taxonomic home for Marburg and Ebola viruses? *Intervirology.* **18** (1–2), 24–32.

Kiley, M.P., Cox, N.J., Elliott, L.H., Sanchez, A., DeFries, R., Buchmeier, M.J., Richman, D.D., and McCormick, J.B. (1988) Physicochemical properties of Marburg virus: evidence for three distinct virus strains and their relationship to Ebola virus. *J. Gen. Virol.* **69** (Pt 8), 1957–1967.

Kindzelskii, A.L., Yang, Z., Nabel, G.J., Todd, R.F. 3rd, and Petty, H.R. (2000) Ebola virus secretory glycoprotein (sGP) diminishes Fc gamma RIIIB-toCR3 proximity on neutrophils. *J. Immunol.* **164** (2), 953–958.

Kissling, R.E., Robinson, R.Q., Murphy, F.A., and Whitfield, S.G. (1968) Agent of disease contracted from green monkeys. *Science.* **160** (830), 888–890.

Knight, S.C. and Macatonia, S.E. (1988) Dendritic cells and viruses. *Immunol. Lett.* **19** (3), 177–181.

Kochneva, G.V., Urmanov, I.H., Ryabchikova, E.I., Streltsov, V.V., and Serpinsky, O.I. (1994) Fine mechanisms of ectromelia virus thymidine kinase-negative mutants avirulence. *Virus Res.* **34** (1), 49–61.

Kolesnikova, L.V., Riabchikova, E.I., Rassadkin, Iu.N., and Grazhdant-seva, A.A. (1997) Ultrastructural stereological analysis of monkey lungs during experimental Ebola fever. *Biull. Eksp. Biol. Med.* **123** (2), 205–208. Russian.

Kolesnikova, L., Muhlberger, E., Ryabchikova, E., and Becker, S. (2000) Ultrastructural organization of recombinant Marburg virus nucleoprotein: comparison with Marburg virus inclusions. *J. Virol.* **74** (8), 3899–3904.

Kolesnikova, L., Bugany, H., Klenk, H.D., and Becker, S. (2002) VP40, the matrix protein of Marburg virus, is associated with membranes of the late endosomal compartment. *J. Virol.* **76** (4), 1825–1838.

Korb, G., Bechtelsheimer, H., and Gegick, P. (1969) Die Morphologie der Leber bei der "Marburg—Virus"—Krankheit. *Modern Gastroenterology.* S.1307–1308.

Kuno, G. and Bailey, R.E. (1994) Cytokine responses to dengue infection among Puerto Rican patients. *Mem. Inst. Oswaldo Cruz.* **89** (2), 179–182.

Le, J.M. and Vilcek, J. (1989) Interleukin 6: a multifunctional cytokine regulating immune reactions and the acute phase protein response. *Lab. Invest.* **61** (6), 588–602.

LeGuenno, B., Formenty, P., Wyers, M., Gounon, P., Walker, F., and Boesch, C. (1995) Isolation and partial characterization of a new strain of Ebola virus. *Lancet.* **345** (8960), 1271–1274.

LeGuenno, B. (1997) Haemorrhagic fevers and ecological perturbations. *Arch. Virol. Suppl.* **13**, 191–199.

Leaver, H.A., Yap, P.L, Rogers, P., Wright, I., Smith, G., Williams, P.E., France, A.J., Craig, S.R., Walker, W.S., and Prescott, R.J. (1995) Peroxides in human leucocytes in acute septic shock: a preliminary study of acute phase changes and mortality. *Eur. J. Clin. Invest.* **25** (10), 777–783.

Leroy, E.M., Baize, S., Volchkov, V.E., Fisher-Hoch, S.P., Georges-Courbot, M.C., Lansoud-Soukate, J., Capron, M., Debre, P., McCormick, J.B., and Georges, A.J. (2000) Human asymptomatic Ebola infection and strong inflammatory response. *Lancet.* **355** (9222), 2210–2215.

Lonigro, A.J., McMurdo, L., Stephenson, A.H., Sprague, R.S., and Weintraub, N.L. (1996) Hypotheses regarding the role of pericytes in regulating movement of fluid, nutrients, and hormones across the microcirculatory endothelial barrier. *Diabetes.* **45** (Suppl. 1), S38–S43.

Lub, M.Iu., Sergeev, A.N., P'iankov, O.V., P'iankova, O.G., Petrishchenko, V.A., and Kotliarov, L.A. (1995) Certain pathogenetic characteristics of a disease in monkeys in infected with the Marburg virus by an airborne route. *Vopr. Virusol.* **40** (4), 158–161. Russian.

Luban, J. (2001) HIV-1 and Ebola virus: The getaway driver nabbed. *Nat. Med.* **7** (12), 1278–1280.

Luchko, S.V., Dadaeva, A.A., Ustinova, E.N., Sizikova, L.P., Riabchikova, E.I., and Sandakhchiev, L.S. (1995) Experimental study of Ebola haemorrhagic fever in baboon models. *Biull. Eksp. Biol. Med.* **120** (9), 302–304. Russian.

Mackay, C.R. (2001) Chemokines: immunology's high impact factors. *Nat. Immunol.* **2** (2), 95–101.

Martini, G.A. (1971) Marburg virus disease: clinical syndrome. *Marburg Virus Disease.* Berlin: Springer-Verlag, 1–9.

Martin-Serrano, J., Zang, T., and Beiniasz, P.D. (2001) HIV-1 and Ebola virus encode small peptide motifs that recruit Tsg101 to sites of particle assembly to facilitate egress. *Nat. Med.* **7** (12), 1313–1319.

Maruyama, T., Rodriguez, L.L., Jahrling, P.B., Sanchez, A., Khan, A.S., Nichol, S.T., Peters, C.J., Parren, P.W., and Burton, D.R. (1999) Ebola virus can be effectively neutralized by antibody produced in natural human infection. *J. Virol.* **73** (7), 6024–6030.

Mayanskii, A.H. (1995) Modern evolution of Mechnikov's idea of intravascular inflammation. *Immunologiya.* (4), 8–14.

McCullough, K.C., Basta, S., Knotig, S., Gerber, H., Schaffner, R., Kim, Y.B., Saalmuller, A., and Summerfield, A. (1999) Intermediate stages in monocyte-macropahge differentiation modulate phenotype and susceptibility to virus infection. *Immunology.* **98** (2), 203–212.

McIntyre, K.W. and Welsh, R.M. (1986) Accumulation of natural killer and cytotoxic T large granular lymphocytes in the liver during virus infection. *J. Exp. Med.* **164** (5), 1667–1681.

McIntyre, K.W., Natuk, R.J., Biron, C.A., et al. (1988) Blastogenesis of large granular lymphocytes in nonlymphoid organs. *J. Leukoc. Biol.* **43** (6), 492–501.

Mena, I., Fischer, C., Gebhard, J.R., Perry, C.M., Harkins, S., and Whitton, J.L. (2000) Coxsackievirus infection of the pancreas: evaluation of receptor expression, pathogenesis, and immunopathology. *Virology.* **271** (2), 276–288.

Miranda, M.E., White, M.E., Dayrit, M.M., Hayes, C.G., Ksiazek, T.G., and Burans, J.P. (1991) Seroepidemiological study of filovirus related to Ebola in the Philippines (Letter). *Lancet.* **337** (8738), 425–426.

MMWR. (1995) Outbreak of Ebola viral hemorrhagic fever - Zaire 1995. *MMWR.* **44** (19), 381–382.

Morvan, J.M., Deubel, V., Gounon, P., Nakoune, E., Barriere, P., Murri, S., Perpete, O., Selekon, B., Couldrier, D., Gautier-Hion, A., Colyn, M., and Volehkov, V. (1999) Identification of Ebola virus sequences present as RNA or DNA in organs of terrestrial small mammals of the Central African Republic. *Microbes Infect.* **1** (14), 1193–11201.

Movat, H.Z. and Wasi, S. (1985) Severe microvascular injury induced by lysosomal releasates of human polymorphonuclear leucocytes. Increase in vasopermeability, hemorrhage, and microthrombosis due to degradation of subendothelial and perivascular matrices. *Amer. J. Pathol.* **121** (3), 404–417.

Movat, H.Z. (1987) Tumor necrosis factor and interleukin-1: role in acute inflammation and microvascular injury. *J. Lab. Clin. Med.* **110** (6), 668–681.

Movat, H. Inflammatory reactions. Amsterdam: Elsevier, 285. p. 365.

Murohara, T., Buerke, M., and Lefer, A.M. (1994) Polymorphonuclear leukocyte-induced vasocontraction and endothelial dysfunction. Role of selectins. *Arterioscler. Thromb.* **14** (9), 1509–1519.

Murphy, F.A., Simpson, D.I., Whitefield, S.G., Zlotnik, I., and Carter, G.B. (1971) Marburg virus infection in monkeys. Ultrastructural studies. *Lab. Invest.* **24** (4), 279–291.

Murphy, F.A., Van der Groen, G., Whitfield, S.G., and Lange, F.V. (1978) Ebola and Marburg virus morphology and taxonomy. In *Ebola virus haemorrhagic fever* (Ed S.R. Pattyn), pp. 61-84. New York: Elsevier North Holland Publishing Co.

Murphy, F.A. (1996) Virus taxonomy. In *Fields Virology* (Eds B.N. Fields, D.M. Knipe, and P.M. Howley), pp. 15–57. Philadelphia: Lippincott-Raven.

Nermut, M.V., Hockley, D.J., and Gelderblom, H. (1987) Electron microscopy: methods for structural analysis of the virion. And electron microscopy: methods for study of virus/cell interaction. In *Animal virus structure. Perspectives in Med. Virol.* 3 (Eds M.V. Nermut and A.C. Steven), pp. 21–60. London: Elsevier, Amsterdam-N.Y.

Nossal, G.J.V., Abbot, A., Mitchell, J., and Lummus, Z. (1968) Antigens in immunity. XV. Ultrastructural features of antigen capture in primary and secondary lymphoid follicles. *J. Exp. Med.* **127** (2), 277–290.

Pease, D.C. (1960) *Histological techniques for electron microscopy.* New York: Acad. Press.

Pereboeva, L.A., Tkachev, V.K., Kolesnikova, L.V., Krendeleva, L.Ia., Riabchikova, E.I., and Smolina, M.P. (1993) The ultrastructural changes in guinea pig organs during the serial passage of the Ebola virus. *Vopr. Virusol.* **38** (4), 179–182. Russian.

Peters, D. and Muller, G. (1969) The Marburg agent and structures associated with leptospira. *Lancet.* **1** (7601), 923–925.

Peters, D., Muller, G., and Slenczka, W. (1971) Morphology, development and classification of the Marburg agent. In *Marburg Virus Disease* (Eds G.A. Martini and R. Siegert), pp. 68–83. Berlin: Springer-Verlag.

Peters, C.J., Johnson, E.D., and McKee, C.K. Jr. (1991) Filoviruses and management of viral hemorrhagic fevers. In *Textbook of human virology* (Ed B. Belshe), pp. 699–712. St. Louis: Mosby Year Book.

Peters, C.J., Sanchez, A., Rollin, P.E., Ksiazek, T.G., and Murphy, F.A. (1996) Filoviridae: Marburg and Ebola Viruses. In *Fields Virology Third Edition* (Eds B.N. Fields, D.M. Knipe, P.M. Howley, et al.), pp. 1161–1176. Philadelphia: Lippincott-Raven Publishers.

Pilaro, A.M., Taub, D.D., McCormick, K.L., Williams, H.M., Sayers, T.J., Fogler, W.E., and Wiltrout, R.H. (1994) TNF-alpha is a principal cytokine involved in the recruitment of NK cells to liver parenchyma. *J. Immunol.* **153** (1), 333–342.

Pinet, V., Malnati, M.S., and Long, E.O. (1994) Two processing pathways for the MHC class II-restricted presentation of exogenous influenza virus antigen. *J. Immunol.* **152** (10), 4852–4860.

Preston, R. (1994) *The Hot Zone.* New York: Random House.

Pringle, C.R. (1997) The order Mononegavirales—current status. *Arch. Virol.* **142** (11), 2321–2326.

ProMed-mail. Ebola Hemorrhagic Fever - Congo Rep: Suspected. ProMed-mail 2003; 5 Feb: 20030205.0315. <http://www.promedmail.org>. Accessed 12 June 2003.

ProMed-mail. Ebola hemorrhagic fever, apes - Congo Rep. (04). ProMed-mail 2003; 4 April: 20030404.0824. <http://www.promedmail.org>. Accessed 12 June 2003.

ProMed-mail. Ebola hemorrhagic fever - Congo Rep. (23). ProMed-mail 2003; 14 April: 20030414.0912. <http://www.promedmail.org>. Accessed 12 June 2003.

Pyankov, O.V., Sergeev, A.N., P'iankova, O.G., and Chepurnov, A.A. (1995) Experimental Ebola fever in Macaca mulatta. *Vopr. Virusol.* **40** (3), 113–115. Russian.

Ratnoff, O.D. and Forbes, Ch.D. (1984) *Disorders of Hemostasis.* New York, W. B. Saunders, 577.

Richards, G.A., Murphy, S., Jobson, R., Mer, M., Zinman, C., Taylor, R., Swanepoel, R., Duse, A., Sharp, G., De La Rey, I.C., and Kassianides, C. (2000) Unexpected Ebola virus in a tertiary setting: clinical and epidemiologic aspects. *Crit. Care Med.* **28** (1), 240–244.

Rippey, J.J., Schepers, N.J., and Gear, J.H. (1976) The pathology of Marburg virus disease. *S. Afr. Med. J.* **66** (2), 50–54.

Risberg, B., Smith, L., and Ortenwall, P. (1991) Oxygen radicals and lung injury. *Acta Anaesthesiol. Scand. Suppl.* (95), 106–118.

Rouse, B.T., Norley, S., and Martin, S. (1988) Antiviral cytotoxic T lymphocyte induction and vaccination. *Rev. Infect. Dis.* **10** (1) 16–33.

Ruiz-Arguello, M.B., Goni, F.M., Pereira, F.B., and Nieva, J.L. (1998) Phosphatidylinositol-dependent membrane fusion induced by a putative fusogenic sequence of Ebola virus. *J. Virol.* **72** (3), 1775–1781.

Ruska, H. (1940) Die Sichtbarmaching der Bacteriophagen Lyse in Ubermikros. *Naturwissenschaften.* **28**, 45–46.

Ryabchikova, E.I., Baranova, S.G., Tkachev, V.K., and Grazhdantseva, A.A. (1993) The morphological changes in Ebola infection in guinea pigs. *Vopr. Virusol.* **38** (4), 176–179. Russian.

Ryabchikova, E.I., Vorontsova, L.A., Skripchenko, A.A., Shestopalov, A.M., and Sandakhchiev, L.S. (1994) Involvement of internal organs of experimental animals infected with Marburg disease virus. *Biull. Eksp. Biol. Med.* **117** (4), 430–434. Russian.

Ryabchikova, E., Kolesnikova, L., Smolina, M., Tkachev, V., Pereboeva, L., Baranova, S., Grazhdantseva, A., and Rassadkin, Y. (1996) Ebola virus infection in guinea pigs: presumable role of granulomatous inflammation in pathogenesis. *Arch. Virol.* **141** (5), 909–921.

Ryabchikova, E., Strelets, L., Kolesnikova, L., Pyankov, O., and Sergeev, A. (1996a) Respiratory Marburg virus infection in guinea pigs. *Arch. Virol.* **141** (11), 2177–2190.

Ryabchikova, E.I., Kolesnikova, L.V., and Rassadkin, Iu. N. (1998) Microscopic study of species specific features of hemostatic impairment in Ebola virus infected monkeys. *Vestn. Ross. Akad. Med. Nauk.* (3), 51–55. Russian.

Ryabchikova, E.I., Kolesnikova, L.V., and Netesov, S.V. (1999) Animal pathology of filoviral infections. *Curr. Top. Microbiol. Immunol.* **235**, 145–173.

Ryabchikova, E.I., Kolesnikova, L.V., and Luchko, S.V. (1999a) An analysis of features of pathogenesis in two animal models of Ebola virus infection. *J. Infect. Dis.* **179** (Suppl. 1), S199–S202.

Ryzhikov, A.B., Ryabchikova, E.I., Sergeev, A.N., and Tkacheva, N.V. (1995) Spread of Venezuelan equine encephalitis virus in mice olfactory tract. *Arch. Virol.* **140** (12), 2243–2254.

Salazar-Mather, T.P., Hamilton, T.A., and Biron, C.A. (2000) A chemokine-to-cytokine-to chemokine cascade critical in antiviral defense. *J. Clin. Invest.* **105** (7), 985–993.

Salyer, J.L., Bohnsack, J.F., Knape, W.A., Shigeoka, A.O., Ashwood, E.R., and Hill, H.R. (1990) Mechanisms of tumor necrosis factor-alpha alteration of PMN adhesion and migration. *Am. J. Pathol.* **136** (4), 831–841.

Salzman, N.H. and Maxfield, F.R. (1989) Fusion accessibility of endocytic compartments along the recycling and lysosomal endocytic pathways in intact cells. *J. Cell Biol.* **109** (5), 2097–2104.

Sanchez, A., Kiley, M.P., Klenk, H.D., and Feldmann, H. (1992) Sequence analysis of the Marburg virus nucleoprotein gene: comparison to Ebola virus and other non-segmented negative strand RNA viruses. *J. Gen. Virol.* **73** (Pt 2), 347–357.

Sanchez, A., Kiley, M.P., Holloway, B.P., and Auperin, D.D. (1993) Sequence analysis of the Ebola virus genome: organization, genetic elements, and comparison with the genome of Marburg virus. *Virus Res.* **29** (3), 215–240.

Sanchez, A., Trappier, S.G., Mahy, B.W., Peters, C.J., and Nichol, S.T. (1996) The virion glycoproteins of Ebola viruses are encoded in two reading frames and are expressed through transcriptional editing. *Proc. Natl. Acad. Sci. USA.* **93** (8), 3602–3607.

Sanger, C., Muhlberger, E., Ryabchikova, E., Kolesnikova, L., Klenk, H.D., and Becker, S. (2001) Sorting of Marburg virus surface protein and virus release take place at opposite surfaces of infected polarized epithelial cells. *J. Virol.* **75** (3), 1274–1283.

Sanger, C., Muhlberger, E., Lotfering, B., Klenk, H.D., and Becker, S. (2002) The Marburg virus surface protein GP is phosphorylated at its ectodomain. *Virology.* **295** (1):20–9.

Sato, T., Selleri, C., Young, N.S., and Maciejewski, J.P. (1995) Hematopoietic inhibition by interferon-gamma is partially mediated through interferon regulatory factor-1. *Blood.* **86** (9), 3373–3380.

Schaeffer, R.C. Jr., Bitrick, M.S. Jr., Connolly, B., Jenson, A.B., and Gong, F. (1993) Pichinde virus-induced respiratory failure due to obstruction of the small airways: structure and function. *Exp. Lung Res.* **19** (6), 715–729.

Schnittler, H.J., Mahner, F., Drenckhahn, D., Klenk, H.D., and Feldmann, H. (1993) Replication of Marburg virus in human endothelial cells. A possible mechanism for the development of viral hemorrhagic disease. *J. Clin. Invest.* **91** (4), 1301–1309.

Schou, S. and Hansen, A.K. (2000) Marburg and Ebola virus infections in laboratory non-human primates: a literature review. *Comp. Med.* **50** (2), 108–123.

Serpinski, O.I., Kochneva, G.V., Urmanov, I.Kh., Sivolobova, G.F., and Riabchikova, E.I. (1996) Construction of recombinant variants or orthopoxviruses by inserting foreign genes into intragenic region of viral genome. *Mol. Biol. (Mosk).* **30** (5), 1055–1065. Russian.

Shalaby, M.R., Aggarwal, B.B., Rinderknecht, E., Svedersky, I.P., Finkle, B.S., and Palladino, M.A. Jr. (1985) Activation of human polymorphonuclear neutrophil functions by interferon-gammas and tumor necrosis factors. *J. Immunol.* **135** (3), 2069–2073.

Siegert, R., Shu, H.L., Slenczka, W. et al. (1967) On the etiology of an unknown human infection originating from monkeys. *Dtsch. Med. Wochenschr.* **92** (51), 2341–2343. German.

Siegert, R., Shu, H.L., and Slenczka, W. (1968) Zur Diagnostik und Pathogenese der Infektion mit Marburg-Virus. *Dtsch. Arzebl.* **65**, 1827–1830.

Siegert, R. (1972) Marburg virus. *Virology monographs.* **11**, 98–153.

Simpson, D.I. (1980) Exotic infectious diseases: Marburg/Ebola/ haemorrhagic fevers. *R. Soc. Health J.* **100** (2), 52–56.

Singh, M., Berger, B., and Kim, P.S. (1999) LearnCoil-VMF: computational evidence for coiled-coil-like motifs in many viral membrane-fusion proteins. *J. Mol. Biol.* **290** (5), 1031–1041.

Skripchenko, A.A., Shestopalov, A.M., and Iaroslavtseva, O.Ia. (1991) A comparative study of the in-vitro interaction of the Marburg virus with macrophages from different animal species. *Vopr. Virusol.* **36** (6), 503–506. Russian.

Skripchenko, A.A., Riabchikova, E.I., Vorontsova, L.A., Shestopalov, A.M., and Viazunov, S.A. (1994) Marburg virus and mononuclear phagocytes: study of interactions. *Vopr. Virusol.* **39** (5), 214–218. Russian.

Smith, C.E., Simpson, D.I., Bowen, E.T., and Zlotnik, I. (1967) Fatal human disease from vervet monkeys. *Lancet.* **2** (7526), 1119–1121.

Smith, J.A. (1994) Neutrophils, host defense, and inflammation: a double-edged sword. *J. Leukoc. Biol.* **56** (6), 672–686.

Steinman, R.M. (1991) The dendritic cell system and its role in immunogenicity. *Annu Rev. Immunol.* **9**, 271–296.

Stroeher, U., West, E., Bugany, H., Klenk, H.D., Schnittler, H.J., and Feldmann, H. (2001) Infection and activation of monocytes by Marburg and Ebola viruses. *J. Virol.* **75** (22), 11025–11033.

Sui, J. and Marasco, W.A. (2002) Evidence against Ebola Virus sGP Binding to Human Neutrophils by a Specific Receptor. *Virology.* **303** (1), 9–14.

Summerfield, A., Knotig, S.M., and McCullough, K.C. (1998) Lymphocyte apoptosis during classical swine fever: implication of activation-induced cell death. *J. Virol.* **72** (3), 1853–1861.

Swanepoel, R., Leman, P.A., Burt, F.J., Zachariades, N.A., Braack, L.E., Ksiazek, T.G., Rollin, P.E., Zaki, S.R., and Peters, C.J. (1996) Experimental inoculation of plants and animals with Ebola virus. *Emerg. Infec. Dis.* **2** (4), 321–325.

Takada, A., Robinson, C., Goto, H., Sanchez, A., Murti, K.G., Whitt, M.A., and Kawaoka, Y. (1997) A system for functional analysis of Ebola virus glycoprotein. *Proc. Natl. Acad. Sci. USA.* **94** (26), 14764–14769.

Takada, A., Watanabe, S., Ito, H., Okazaki, K., Kida, H., and Kawaoka, Y. (2000) Downregulation of beta1 integrins by Ebola virus glycoprotein: implication for virus entry. *Virology.* **278** (1), 20–26.

Taub, D.D. and Oppenheim, J.J. (1994) Chemokines, inflammation and the immune system. *Ther. Immunol.* **1** (4), 229–246.

Teodoro, J.G. and Branton, P.E. (1997) Regulation of apoptosis by viral gene products. *J. Virol.* **71** (3), 1739–1746.

Thelen, M., Dewald, B. and Baggiolini, M. (1993) Neutrophil signal transduction and activation of the respiratory burst. *Physiol. Rev.* **73**(4):797-821

US Government Printing Office (1999). *Biosafety in Microbiological and Biomedical Laboratories (BMBL) 4th Edition*, Washington.

Virus Taxonomy. *Seventh Report of International Committee of Taxonomy of Viruses* (Eds M.H.V. van Regenmortel, C.M. Fauquet, D.H.L. Bishop, E.B. Carstens, M.K. Estes, S.M. Lemon, J. Maniloff, M.A. Mayo, D.J. McGeoch, C.R. Pringle, and R.B. Wickner).

Volchkov, V.E., Blinov, V.M., and Netesov, S.V. (1992) The envelope glycoprotein of Ebola virus contains an immunosuppressive-like domain similar to oncogenic retroviruses. *FEBS Lett.* **305** (3), 181–184.

Volchkov, V.E., Becker, S., Volchkova, V.A., Ternovoj, V.A., Kotov, A.N., Netesov, S.V., and Klenk, H.D. (1995) GP mRNA of Ebola virus is edited by the Ebola virus polymerase and by T7 and vaccinia virus polymerases. *Virology.* **214** (2), 421–430.

Volchkov, V., Volchkova, V., Eckel, C., Klenk, H.D., Bouloy, M., LeGuenno, B., and Feldmann, H. (1997) Emergence of subtype Zaire Ebola virus in Gabon. *Virology.* **232** (1), 139–144

Volchkov, V.E., Volchkova, V.A., Slenczka, W., Klenk, H.D., and Feldmann, H. (1998) Release of viral glycoproteins during Ebola virus infection. *Virology.* **245** (1), 110–119.

Weissenhorn, W., Calder, L.J., Wharton, S.A., Skehel, J.J., and Wiley, D.C. (1998) The central structural feature of the membrane fusion protein subunit from the Ebola virus glycoprotein is a long triple-stranded coiled coil. *Proc. Natl. Acad. Sci. USA.* **95** (11), 6032–6036.

Williams, R.C. (1953) The shapes and sizes of purified viruses as determined by electron microscopy. *Proc. Cold Spring Harb. Symp. Quant. Biol.* **18**, 185–196.

Wilson, J.A., Hevey, M., Bakken, R., Guest, S., Bray, M., Schmaljohn, A.L., and Hart, M.K. (2000) Epitopes involved in antibody-mediated protection from Ebola virus. *Science.* **287** (5458), 1664–1666.

Witko-Sarsat, V., Rieu, P., Descamps-Latscha, B., Lesavre, P., and Halbwachs-Mecarelli, L. (2000) Neutrophils: molecules, functions and pathophysiological aspects. *Lab Invest.* **80** (5), 617–653.

Wool-Lewis, R.J. and Bates, P. (1998) Characterization of Ebola virus entry by using pseudotyped viruses: identification of receptor-deficient cell lines. *J. Virol.* **72** (4), 3155–3160.

Wool-Lewis RJ, Bates P. (1999) Endoproteolytic processing of the ebola virus envelope glycoprotein: cleavage is not required for function. *J. Virol.* **73** (2),1419–26.

World Health Organization (WHO). (1978) Ebola haemorrhagic fever in Sudan, 1976. *Bull World Health Organ.* **56** (2), 247–270.

World Health Organization (WHO). (1978a) Ebola haemorrhagic fever in Zaire, 1976. *Bull World Health Organ.* **56** (2), 271–293.

World Health Organization (WHO) Scientific Group. (1985) Arthropod-borne and rodent-borne viral diseases. *WHO Technical Report Series 1985.* **719**, 1–116.

World Health Organization (WHO). (1996) Outbreak of Ebola haemorrhagic fever in Gabon officially declared over. *Weekly Epidemiol. Rec.* **71**, 125–126.

World Health Organization (WHO). (2002) "Disease Outbreaks: Ebola haemorrhagic fever" *Communicable Disease Surveillance and Response Disease Outbreak News.* <http://www.who.int/disease-outbreak-news/disease/A98.4.htm> (27 May 2003).

Yang, K.D., Lee, C.S., Hwang, K.P., Chu, M.L., and Shaio, M.F. (1995) A model to study cytokine profiles in primary and heterologously secondary Dengue-2 virus infections. *Acta Virol.* **39** (1), 19–21.

Yang, Z., Delgado, R., Xu, L., Todd, R.F., Nabel, E.G., Sanchez, A., and Nabel, G.J. (1998) Distinct cellular interactions of secreted and transmembrane Ebola virus glycoproteins. *Science.* **279** (5353), 1034–1037.

Yang, Z.Y., Duckers, H.J., Sullivan, N.J., Sanchez, A., Nabel, E.G., and Nabel, G.J. (2000) Identification of the Ebola virus glycoprotein as the main viral determinant of vascular cell cytotoxicity and injury. *Nat. Med.* **6** (8), 886–889.

Zaki, S.R., Goldsmith, C.R., Greer, P.W., Coffield, L.M., Rollin, P.E., Callain, P., Khan, A.S., Ksiazek, T.G., and Peters, C.J. (1995) Pathology of Ebola virus hemorrhagic fever, Kikwit, Zaire. *J. Infect. D is.*

Zaki, S.R. and Kilmarx, P.H. (1997) Ebola virus hemorrhagic fever. In *Pathology of Emerging Infections* (Eds C.R. Horsburgh and A.M. Nelson), pp. 299–312. Am. Soc. Microbiol., Washington.

Zlotnik, I. (1969) Marburg agent disease: pathology. *Trans. R. Soc. Trop. Med. Hyg.* **63** (3), 310–327.

Index

Page numbers followed by "F" mean that the information appears in the figure. Page numbers followed by "T" mean that the information appears in the table.

F = figure; T = table

F = figure; T = table

F = figure; T = table

F = figure; T = table